FAMILY-BASED TREATMENT IN COMMUNICATIVE DISORDERS

A SYSTEMIC APPROACH

JAMES R. ANDREWS, PH.D.
Professor
Department of Communicative Disorders
Northern Illinois University
DeKalb, Illinois

MARY A. ANDREWS, M.S.
Couple & Family Therapist
Private Practice
DeKalb, Illinois

D1545187

JANELLE PUBLICATIONS, INC.
DeKalb, IL 60115

Copyright© 2000, Janelle Publications, Inc.
P.O. Box 811   DeKalb, IL 60115

Printed in the United States of America.
ISBN 1-890265-03-9

CONTENTS

PROLOGUE

The first edition of Family-Based Treatment in Communicative Disorders broke new ground by ushering Speech and Language Pathologists into an era of considering the family as a unit of change in our therapeutic process. For many of us, this book changed our perspective on treatment of speech and language disorders and enabled us to increase the speed and efficiency with which therapeutic changes could be accomplished. The first edition was seminal in that it also provided one of the first methodologies for treating communication skills in a naturalistic context as opposed to attempting to "teach speech or language skills" in the vacuum of a clinician's therapy room. However, just as important, the Andrews' family based approach to speech language pathology provided an approach that enhances the satisfaction derived from the clinical process, both for the clinician and the client(s) we serve. As I began to incorporate Andrews and Andrews' principles into my own practice I was amazed and delighted at the positive responses to the intervention I began receiving from my families. Family members often expressed their delight at, "being taken seriously," and showed a renewed enthusiasm for working with their loved-one in realistic communication settings.

For those readers who are approaching this revised volume as your first introduction to Andrews and Andrews, I envy you. You will discover a means of treatment that will significantly enhance your clinical skills and your enjoyment of the clinical process, no matter how long you have been practicing. The way the authors intertwine case studies throughout their discussions of concepts and treatment techniques, makes their writing a pleasure to read and effortless to retain. We all can identify with their examples, and take solace in the recognition that these two authors are actual clinicians, who understand first hand the issues we all face in the clinical world.

For others of you, who have read and implemented the approaches in the first edition, I know you will appreciate the new insights and techniques this volume provides. For example, chapter four introduces a new technique called "scaling" that enables a clinician to help a family observe and quantify communicative changes as they occur. For many of us, enabling a family to see a client's communication growth in a realistic way is one of the great challenges we face. Other techniques introduced in this volume are "questioning" and "use of self." Chapter six provides new methods for helping families assess the effectiveness of clinical methods and adapt their goals and assignments according to new information gleaned from each session. The authors have also added a new discussion of family based treatment as it directly applies to early-intervention in the ninth chapter. Finally, the last chapter provides a discussion that will be welcome to all of us, on how to work with challenging family situations.

The second edition of Family-Based Treatment in Communicative Disorders is a welcome addition to all professional libraries. Students of speech-language pathology and seasoned clinicians alike will find it an invaluable resource of methods and practical techniques for enhancing communication skills in the real world.

Martha S. Burns, Ph.D.
Adjunct Associate Professor
Northwestern University
Evanston, Illinois
Senior Clinical Specialist
Scientific Learning Corporation
Berkeley, California

ACKNOWLEDGMENTS

We cannot fully express our gratitude to the hundreds of families with whom we have worked. Each of them has taught us something new and all of them have encouraged us as they faithfully attended sessions, disagreed with some of our "strange" ideas, followed through on our suggestions, and became enabled partners in creating speech-language change. They have been wonderful resources for us and for their family members with communicative disorders.

None of our work would be possible without the consistent, collegial support of the faculty and staff of the Department of Communicative Disorders at Northern Illinois University. They have supported us in every way possible in spite of our departure from the traditional medical model. We especially thank Gip Seaver, Chair of the Department, whose unfailing good humor makes our work fun, and Anne Davidson, supervisor extraordinaire, whose clinical ability and gentle style has expanded our horizons in unexpectedly productive ways.

Our graduate students at Northern Illinois University have made our work with families incredibly enjoyable. Their commitment to the systemic paradigm before and after graduation; their superb ability to join with families and facilitate speech-language change; their willingness to challenge us with new ideas; and their laughter, when our jokes are funny and even when they are not-so funny, has invigorated us to continue our work. And, what a privilege it has been to teach graduate students from the University of Alberta who encouraged us immensely as they put Family-Based Treatment into practice. Thank you all for energizing and motivating us to continue our work.

Other friends from throughout North America have supported us by sharing their family-centered treatment ideas and remarkable professional lives with us. Thank you Robin Alvares, University of Edinboro; Margaret Briggs, Seton Hall University; Ellen Dodge, Phillips Brooks School, Menlo Park, California; Susan Riley, University of Maine; and Liz Webster, Glenrose Rehabilitation Hospital, Edmonton, Alberta, Canada. We appreciate, enjoy, and respect you all!

As in the first edition, a word about our own family is in order. Our time with them is our therapy as they bring laughter, love and wisdom into our lives. Dave, has recycled from a degree in music to a degree in speech-language pathology and now works for the Portland Early Intervention Program. Sarah, his wife, is a Montessori educator. Sarah and Dave have given us our beautiful grandsons, Julian and Evan. Tim is completing a masters degree in special education and plans to specialize in work with children having autism. Mark has finished a degree in sociology and is working in the

Portland Early Intervention Program as an assistant in a supportive integrated classroom. Donna, his wife, uses her English/computer skills while working for a book company. If we had been lucky enough to have daughters, they could not have been more perfect than our two wonderful daughters-in-law. Our growing family continues to show us, in remarkably creative ways, the power of the family.

INTRODUCTION
TO
THE SECOND EDITION

Family-Based Treatment is a systemic, solution-focused, family-centered model for providing speech-language services that integrates counseling techniques with assessment and treatment. The model is based on a blend of principles and techniques of speech-language pathology and family therapy which we have developed and used with a wide variety of families in the last seventeen years. This book describes the model and illustrates its use through case studies. All of the case studies describe families with whom we have worked. In every case, however, names and details have been changed to protect confidentiality.

We have used the Family-Based Treatment model and taught it to graduate students in classes and practicum since we began developing it in 1982. Since the first edition was published, we have added new information and techniques to our practice. Solution-focused treatment, for example is a family therapy approach from which we have borrowed and now routinely integrate with our work with families having members with communicative delays or disorders. Most of the solution-focused principles and techniques we now use were not available at the time of the first edition of this book. In addition, family-centered treatment has become standard practice in early intervention since we first described Family-Based Treatment. As the details of family-centered treatment evolved, we happily realized that what was being described was very close to the model we were using and advocating.

Like the first edition, one of our goals was to write a book for practicing speech-language pathologists that was stimulating, interesting to read, and that offered practical suggestions, some of which could be selected, adapted, and used by the reader in his or her professional context. Not everyone who wants to work with families practices in a setting that permits this to the extent that we describe it. Few, if any, will do it exactly in the manner that we do. It is expected that the approach will be adapted to the reader's clinical situation and that selected parts of the process and some of the techniques will be used as the reader relates to families in the manner most appropriate and feasible. We believe that such a clinician will find that his or her practice of the profession is enriched and that a fascinating profession is made even more so when the influence of families on clients and speech-language change is appreciated and utilized. A second goal, is to introduce the model to students preparing to practice the profession of speech-language pathology. We know from experience that students can become proficient in using the model. We have been highly impressed with the graduate students

1

with whom we have worked as they developed confidence and comfort in working with families. Predictably, their expertise in identifying and using family resources to create positive speech-language change often exceeds ours.

Some new features of this edition are the addition of a chapter on working with challenging family situations (Chapter 12), a significant expansion of principles and techniques for applying the model to early intervention services (Chapter 9), a re-written chapter on assessing the effectiveness of treatment (Chapter 6), a description of additional counseling techniques that may be integrated in treatment (Chapter 8), and the use of the solution-focused technique of scaling that enhances family members' abilities to set long and short-term goals for their child (Chapter 4). Additional new information is infused in each chapter in the book.

If you already use parts of the Family-Based Treatment model, we believe you will find new applications as you read this revised edition of the original book. If you are interested in working with families but have not yet begun, we hope this revision will give you information that encourages you to start. If you are a student preparing to practice the profession, and are learning the individual medical model in most of your classes and practicum we suggest that you consider using a systemic paradigm as a base. Systemic thinking accommodates medical model thinking far better than the medical model can accommodate systemic practice.

We hope that some of the joy we find in working with families is evident to the reader of this book. Nothing in my (Jim) 35 years of experience in the profession has been as stimulating and rewarding as developing, using, and teaching the Family-Based Treatment model.

Jim & Mary Andrews

CHAPTER 1

THE SYSTEMIC PERSPECTIVE

Family members can be a significant resource for change. Speech-language pathologists and audiologists, knowing this, have made various attempts over the years to include parents in treatment. These efforts, until recently, have nearly always been based on the assumptions and framework of the linear (individual) treatment model. Mothers, for example, have been enlisted to carry out structured therapy plans, in effect, assuming the role of an aide working under strict supervision of the speech-language pathologist. The individual continues to be the unit of treatment in this case, but the treatment plan is implemented by someone other than the clinician. More routinely, speech-language pathologists attempt to extend their influence by asking family members to practice words, sentences, etc. with clients much in the same way that physicians give prescriptions to patients. Compliance with the speech-language pathologist's assignments becomes an issue in some cases, and families may be cast in the role of being "uncooperative." Other attempts to involve families are educational in nature. Family members are told about speech-language and hearing problems to inform them about the nature of these disorders. Brochures are available to describe aphasia, cleft palate, language delay, stuttering, and other communicative disorders. All of these efforts are logical and useful extensions of services offered within a linear model. Within that approach, the most significant changes in communicative behavior occur during sessions with the speech-language pathologist. These changes may be enhanced by family cooperation and understanding, but participation of families is secondary to the role of the professional.

While the traditional model continues to be satisfactory in some clinical situations, a desire to enlarge the focus of treatment beyond the direct efforts of speech-language pathologists has emerged. In the 1980's, Frassinelli, et al. (1983), Garbee (1982), Manolson (1985), Neidecker (1987), Superior & Lelchook (1986), Williams (1986), and others suggested that the responsibility for changing communicative behavior may be shared with other significant people in clients' lives and that change might even occur more rapidly and efficiently if this were done. In the 1990's, it became routine for speech-language pathologists to provide classroom-based interventions and to team with teachers, psychologists, social workers, and other school-based personnel. Ellis, Schlaudecker, and Regimbal (1995), for example, describe a collaborative consultation approach in which a speech-language pathologist teamed with a university faculty member, a classroom teacher, and a physical education teacher to teach basic concepts to children of kindergarten age.

The role of families in intervention is highlighted by Bruce, DiVenere, and Bergeron (1998) who state that speech-language pathologists are "in the midst of a transition from the 'expert' model of intervention to forming partnerships with families and serving as resources." (p. 85). The importance of family participation is magnified when we think of offering services to infants and toddlers for whom the traditional individual model seems particularly inappropriate. In their review of the relationship between communication disorders and socioemotional issues, Prizant and Meyer (1993) state that "A family systems perspective is currently viewed as essential for speech-language pathologists working with infants and young children" (p. 62). We couldn't agree more.

While the assumptions of a linear paradigm may be effective when providing traditional individual services, these assumptions are incompatible with services that are collaborative in nature. A shift to a systemic understanding of treatment is a prerequisite to involving families or other professionals successfully in the habilitation/rehabilitation process.

A PARADIGM SHIFT

In order to establish partnerships with families and involve them successfully in the treatment process, it is necessary to change from a linear to a systemic way of thinking about treatment. This challenging and stimulating change in perspective may be referred to as a paradigm shift. As a clinician's view is altered in the direction of systemic thinking, a changed perception affects the manner in which *her professional expertise is used. For example, as she begins to view the interactions that occur between a client and the various members of the client's family as significant for understanding the speech-language-hearing disorder and developing a treatment plan, she likely will want to invite those family members to participate in the treatment process in an active manner.

* Female and male designators will be used alternately throughout the book.

Five of the changes in thinking that we believe support the development of partnerships and significantly impact the way the clinician provides services are a shift from "one truth" to "many truths," from an either/or orientation to a both/and orientation, from labeling behaviors to identifying interactive patterns, from a problem-focus to a solution-focus, and from linear cause-effect change to systems transformation.

From One Truth to Many Truths

The phrase "polyocular view" has been used by deShazer (1985) to describe a situation in which many different interpretations of the same phenomenon are received and accepted as true. As in the adage, two heads are better than one, the combined resources of many eyes (polyocular) generate a view that offers more options for change than that of the one-eyed perspective. Similarly, sound (music in particular) takes on a new dimension as several tracks are superimposed to create a relational whole that is different from the sound generated by one track alone. The sound tracks may be complimentary or dissonant when combined, but each by itself is an accurate representation of its own tune.

Each of the people who interact with an individual having a communication problem has a view of the problem that is influenced by the particular perspective or orientation of that person as well as by the way in which his observations/interactions affect the phenomenon under consideration (e.g., the client's speech-language, the client's behavior, the family as a whole, and family members individually). If we think of truth, in this situation, as something that is held by the observer or that lies within and is created by each observer's view of reality, it becomes natural and useful to learn the perspective of each family member. In other words, in this situation, we think of truth not so much as one particular element or reality to be searched for, determined, and labeled but rather that truth consists of the meaning that each person attributes to the situation. In this view, truth is determined by each person on the basis of his experiences, including those experiences of interacting with the family member of concern. The speech-language pathologist determines her truth about the situation as she learns from the family and assesses the member with a potential communication disorder. Her perspective becomes one of several truths, each one of which is valid and useful as options for contextual treatment are selected. Further, as the clinician and family interact and problem-solve together, the combined perspectives may introduce what Bateson (1979) called "news of difference." In other words, the process of discussing and accepting each perspective and adding it to the "mix," may lead to new thinking about the situation. This evolving new perception, or even new perceptions, may lead to a surprisingly creative array of treatment possibilities that would never have occurred if the clinician had not made the shift from one truth to many truths.

An example of this may be seen in a situation Jim encountered in which the mother's view of her child was that he was too stubborn to talk. The father's view was that the child would talk when he reached the age of four, just as his wife's brother had done. Jim's view was that the child had developmental apraxia and was struggling to speak but couldn't. We agreed to accept each person's view and developed suggestions for each person to carry out that fit his or her reality: the child *can't* talk, he *won't* talk (i.e., he refuses), but he *will* talk. This was "news of difference" for all of us, and a treatment plan in which we could all participate effectively was developed (Andrews & Andrews, 1995). Assuming a polyocular perspective also served to seal a strong partnership that weathered the ups and downs of successes and disappointments along the way toward significant communicative changes for both the child and family.

From Either/Or to Both/And

The polyocular view naturally requires that the clinician adopt a both/and orientation. This is the idea that two or more beliefs, assessments, or observations, though different can be correct. For example, if the mother in a family is very structured, organized and concrete in her view of child rearing and requires orderly behavior from her children while the father is playful, relaxed, and spontaneous with few structured expectations, the children are doubly fortunate because two very useful styles are being modeled and encouraged. This both/and view of two different parenting styles releases resources that will enhance the children's development. If, however, an either/or orientation is adopted by the parents (and children), they are likely to challenge one another about the correctness of each perspective. This challenge will result in a conflict that may banish one of the parenting truths to a covert position in the family's relational style. This either/or conflict diminishes the range of options that are available to those fortunate families that adopt a both/and perspective.

When the clinician adopts a polyocular view, which includes a both/and orientation, she recognizes that her professional perspective regarding treatment is as correct as each family member's view of the problem. An important variable must be added, however. In a family, parents need to accept responsibility for organizing differences so that family life is enhanced. The parents may need to choose situations that are more appropriate for orderly control than for spontaneous play and teach these differences to their children. Or, one parent may need to approach the other in order to discuss these differences and reach consensus about how to manage them. The possibilities are numerous, and the both/and view requires friendly cooperation in order to facilitate optimum use of different, yet valid, opinions. In like manner, the professional must accept responsibility for organizing the variety of views expressed by everyone involved so that the treatment climate is enhanced. It is not sufficient simply to explore different viewpoints and then proceed in a typical linear fashion as though such a discussion had never taken place. Rather, the different views have to be managed to influence new thinking that results in an idiosyncratic treatment plan, framed in the language and expressions of a new perspective. This may be as simple as leading an open, honest, friendly discussion of the differences expressed and by deciding which viewpoints can be most effectively accessed for change to occur.

From Labeling Behaviors to Identifying Interactive Patterns

Most clinicians, when meeting a client and his family members for the first time, think about assessing the problem, describing the communicative characteristics observed, and offering the client and family a diagnosis, or name, for the particular type speech-language-hearing disorder exhibited by the client. Sometimes this diagnosis is determined relatively easily as in most cases of adult stuttering, language delay secondary to hearing loss or cognitive impairment, or hypernasal speech due to velopharyngeal insufficiency. At other times, the diagnosis is more elusive as, for example, when the clinician is confronted with a child who is late to talk and has a history that includes middle ear infections; a child with unintelligible speech; a child whose cooperation is very difficult to elicit; or a client who has a mixed functional-organic communicative disorder.

In some cases, we have observed professionals so concerned about finding a diagnosis that the client's strengths were ignored, and the search for solutions was delayed until additional referrals could be made and the results of the assessments of other professionals were available. Treatment in these cases seemingly could not progress until a label had been applied. In these situations, it seems that our profession's focus on disorders and our adherence to the medical model points us in the direction of seeking ever more information in order to label problems rather than toward beginning the process of treatment and change which, in itself, may later assist in labeling the disorder.

When the diagnosis is elusive or several different diagnoses are offered, we believe that it is wise for the clinician to temporarily abandon her efforts to name the disorder and, instead, begin to explore interactive patterns in order to gather more data about possibilities for treatment. As the clinician and family conduct this exploration and establish a partnership, the nature of the problem and its name may become clearer, or the need for a label may diminish in importance. Further, when a diagnosis must be put on paper because this is required of the clinician, the label often is a metaphor for the problem that may, in fact, have no useful name.

Consider a family that includes a fifteen-year-old daughter. On a particular day in January this girl's behavior is labeled by Mother as "grouchy" and by Grandma as "sullen." Her boyfriend says she's "upset," and her girlfriend worries that she's "depressed." Each of these labels is interesting and is viewed as true by the person expressing concern, but is of limited usefulness in exploring possible solutions to the discomfort shown by the teenager. If a friend of Mother asks questions such as, "How does your daughter show you her 'grouchiness'?"; "What do you do in response?"; "Who else seems to notice that your daughter is upset?"; "How does that person respond?", etc. the mother and friend begin to uncover events that place the "grouchiness" in an interactive context. This interactive understanding of "grouchy behavior" will lead to possibilities for change more efficiently than will the tacit acceptance of the label, "grouchy."

Similarly, when the clinician adopts a systemic perspective, it is natural to shift the focus from a primary concern of finding a label to an exploration of the interactive nature of the problem. Questions such as, "How does Timmy let you know what he wants?", "How do you respond when this happens?"; "Who else seems to be concerned?"; "How does that person respond?", "What's happening during the times when Timmy communicates best?", etc. open the discussion to interactive exploration. The clinician, client, and family members will then begin to discover new possibilities for change. The process also often leads to a fuller understanding of the situation as well as to evolving, natural discussions about possible causes and labels as the clinician-family partnership becomes stronger. (A detailed description of the use of questions in exploring interactive patterns is found in Chapter 8.)

From a Problem Focus to a Solution Focus

When the clinician, client, and family explore the interactive events that surround a communicative disorder, the focus of treatment moves in the direction of solutions. Sometimes new solutions are created. Often, solutions are already a part of the client's and family's behavioral repertoire and simply need to be unearthed and actuated by the clinician.

In Mary's family therapy practice, for example, a family was concerned because their fourteen-year-old son was "lazy." Exploration of the problem revealed that this "laziness" was shown most clearly during times the son was supposed to be doing homework. Further exploration revealed that there were many times when the son did not show "laziness" but showed behaviors that his parents labeled "energetic." These behaviors were associated with his basketball playing, snacking, and guitar playing. Since it was determined that the son was not a "lazy boy," but one who needed to learn to show his energetic behavior in another area of his life, the focus of the family shifted toward helping him apply his energy to homework completion. When the family shifted their view to a solution focus, this freed the boy to recognize and use his abilities differently.

Similarly, as a clinician shifts her focus toward uncovering and creating solutions, the clinician and the family are likely to find unexpected resources that can be used to treat the speech-language-hearing problem. While exploring the interaction surrounding a young child showing signs of pervasive developmental disorder, for example, the parents and clinician may discover that there are times when the child looks at his parents and makes lip movements in response to his mother saying, "Mama." At these times, the parents may notice that they are speaking quietly and slowly to one another, that they are less likely to ask the child questions or to name things, and that the child is rested and in a good mood. These behaviors may be a partial solution to creating an environmental context in which the child is more likely than usual to attend to his parents. When focused on solutions, the systemic clinician creates a climate that facilitates positive communicative changes in clients.

The boy who is seen as "energetic" instead of "lazy" is more likely to do his homework. The parents who are seen as "sensitive" and "creative" are more likely to be successful in helping their family member who has a communicative disorder than those who are viewed as "uncaring" and "inept." When the clinician adopts a solution focus, greater use can be made of the positive resources available within the family system (O'Hanlon & Weiner-Davis, 1989; Walter & Peller, 1992; Berg (1994), and family members become confident and competent in their ability to participate as team members.

From Cause-Effect Change to System Transformation

Most clinicians think of change in a cause-effect way. For example, the clinician first identifies a problem: "articulation of speech was limited to bilabial, tongue tip-alveolar, and glottal sounds. The latter place of articulation was overused with glottal stops being substituted for many voiceless consonants" (Andrews & Andrews, 1986a, p. 410). With this assessment in mind, goals are set and treatment proceeds. Often there seems to be a direct cause-effect relationship between changes in the client's speech and the clinician's implementation of specific treatment strategies. However, many clients report other unexpected changes that seem to be related to the speech-language change but cannot be linked to the treatment process in a linear cause-effect way. Changes such as "he's talking more," "he's more demanding," and "he stands up for himself" are typical of those reported by clients and/or their family members but are not specifically related to treatment efforts to "eliminate the use of glottal stops being substituted for many voiceless consonants." The clinician, client, and family sense, however, that these behavioral changes are associated with the speech-language treatment process. These changes may be said to result from a system transformation (Tomm, 1984).

When working with families, the clinician will experience both system transformation and cause-effect changes. As the speech-language-hearing difficulty is assessed and as the family is respectfully included in that process, the family is likely to transform itself in ways that cannot always be predicted by the clinician. Often these changes are unexpected and are associated with speech-language improvement.

As we worked with T. (age 4), his mother, father, and three siblings, we and the family decided together to use the family's resources to help T. become more intelligible (Andrews & Andrews, 1986a). After fourteen sessions over a nine-month period, T.'s intelligibility had improved nearly 100%, and our services were terminated. During that process, the family had transformed itself in many surprising ways. Formerly, they had been labeled by the professional community as "uncooperative" because they were failing to keep appointments and not following through with treatment recommendations. Near the end of Family-Based Treatment, T.'s kindergarten teacher reported that he looked different, was more kempt, and that his mother had become interested in his work and was eager to cooperate with classroom goals. His formerly unintelligible speech was reported to be completely intelligible in every context. This was confirmed by his second grade teacher, two years later, when she expressed surprise when informed that T. had once had a speech problem. Other changes occurred which likely continue to reverberate in the family system in unexpected and surprising ways.

None of these changes could be linked in a linear fashion to a specific cause. Even the speech-language change could not be specifically linked to our work with the family nor could the change be specifically linked to the competent, involved mother, or the quiet, controlled father, or the teasing brothers, or the nurturing sister. The family had transformed itself in a way that was coherent with their idiosyncratic style (Dell, 1982), and these changes had impacted many areas of T.'s life.

It would have been very difficult to study the 28 sets of interactions occurring among the eight people involved in treatment. Even if this were possible, the reductionist view of "what happened" could not fully reveal the systemic transformations that occurred in a co-evolutionary manner over time. Rather, the family system was accessed in a way that freed its members to take charge of change in their own idiosyncratic way. This included their desire to use the expertise of the clinicians who worked with them.

FOUR SYSTEMIC PRINCIPLES

Family-Based Treatment is a systemic model for providing family-centered speech-language services. The shifts in thinking described above, along with four systemic principles described below, provide the theoretical foundation for the model.

First, *one part of the family cannot be understood in isolation from the rest of the system* (Epstein & Bishop, 1981). The behavior of each family member can be understood more completely when it is experienced relative to the patterns, beliefs, and customs of the family as a whole than when it is analyzed in isolation. Most everyone has had the experience of gaining insights into the behavior of a friend upon being introduced to that person's family of origin. Behaviors of the individual are understood differently in that context. It is traditional in our society for young couples anticipating a serious relationship to meet one another's families. We can assume that many insights have been gleaned through such meetings. While the ostensible purpose may be for the family to meet and evaluate the offspring's friend, the larger amount of information and perhaps the greater evaluation may fall to the "intended" upon seeing the potential mate in the interactive environment of his/her family of origin.

Similarly, the details of a communicative disorder are comprehended in a different way when the clinician views the client in the environment of his family rather than when evaluating and treating the individual alone. In the family context the communicative behavior of the client may be observed relative to the interactions of the entire system. Some families with whom we have worked have had one or two members who were very articulate and verbal, but the child with a language delay had few opportunities to talk. In other cases, family members were so quiet and independent that the child with a language delay, like the rest of the family, rarely sought or received interactive attention. We are not suggesting that there is anything "wrong" with these or other interactive behaviors we have observed in families, nor do we discuss what we observe with families in other than a neutral and accepting manner. Given a communicative disorder, however, those interactive patterns that appear to be facilitative of change may be reinforced and expanded, and those that seem to be perpetuating the problem may be discussed and altered. The information that contextual observation yields is rich, not only for describing the problem, but for developing interventions for change.

Second, *the parts of a family are interrelated; change in one part influences change in other parts of the system* (Epstein & Bishop, 1981). Most everyone who is part of a family has experienced the results of one person being sick with the flu and incapacitated for a day or two. The effects of even a temporary illness such as this are not limited to the person who is ill; everyone in the family is affected. The specific manner in which the lives of the different family members are touched varies with idiosyncratic family patterns, the roles of family members, and the developmental stage of the family. It is not difficult to imagine the varying effects of illness to a father, mother, or young child in a family with pre-school and school-age children. While the specifics are different, it is no less a matter of reacting when one member of a senior citizen couple is ill. When one member of a family is out of town, in trouble, happy, depressed, angry, etc., the behavior of everyone else in the family is influenced, and everyone reacts in some way. One needs only to consider different situations in her own family to appreciate the complex nature of overt and covert reactions and interactions that might accompany a change in one individual.

Similarly, when one member of a family has a communicative disorder, the behavior of all other family members is affected, and all members react. Some typical reactions we have observed include asking the adult with aphasia many questions; asking a child to name pictures and objects; showing anger and embarrassment over a family member's speech disorder; rewarding the verbalizations of a child with delayed language; helping the person with a head injury by saying the words he appeared to be wanting to say; and exaggerating the consonants for the young child with a repaired cleft palate. Obviously, some family reactions facilitate desirable change more than others. When family members of a young child who stuttered modified their behavior to ask fewer questions and reduce the amount of educational instruction they were providing, the child's ability to control his fluency increased. In another family, inattentiveness combined with very limited communicative attempts by the child were part of a family interactive system in which Mom and nine-year-old daughter both talked a lot while Dad was extremely quiet. When the verbal output of the two more talkative family members was reduced, both the child and his father began to speak more. When family members are an integral part of assessment and treatment and are given techniques for reinforcing appropriate communicative behavior, services are not limited to time spent with the clinician, and carryover is enhanced from the outset (Andrews & Andrews, 1986b).

Family members also react to speech-language improvement of their members. The brothers and sisters of a child with unintelligible speech described him as "meaner" and "bossy" after his intelligibility improved and he spoke more. His parents interpreted this behavior as "standing up for himself" and as showing assertiveness verbally rather than physically (Andrews & Andrews, 1986a). The parents of this same child were reported by other social service professionals to be more cooperative. The teacher indicated that the child was dressed better at school and had more friends, and his parents reported that his grades improved. Many changes accompanied an improvement in this child's speech intelligibility.

When a communicative disorder is associated with permanent disability, the effects of that disability extend beyond the daily activities of the immediate family members. Grandparents, great-grandparents, and all extended family members are affected by the disability in ways that permeate their lives throughout the life span. The disability may be known at birth, may become known as the child matures, or may occur later in the life of the individual. Each family member and professional working with the client is profoundly affected by this unexpected event or change.

Third, *transactional patterns of the family shape the behavior of family members* (Epstein & Bishop, 1981). Every individual is affected by the immediate and long ranging family events that shape and form the life experience. The pull of the family system is felt by clinicians and clients alike as they work for speech-language improvement. The speech-language pathologist's awareness of some of these influences may be used to help families promote change in their member who is communicatively disordered. Some of these transactional patterns can be observed by attending to interactions during family sessions; others can be accessed through careful questioning and tracking of behavioral sequences. Some are revealed over time as family members and the clinician become better acquainted; others will remain unknown both to the family and to the clinician.

Complex interactions related to a speech-language problem are likely to include both verbal and non-verbal repetitive patterns among family members. For example, the noisy, messy eating of a teenager with dysarthria evoked admonitions and advice from his mother. Younger brother reacted to the conversation by becoming silent, and Dad responded to all of this with anger at both his wife and the teenager. The teenager in turn ate faster and, therefore, messier and noisier. This pattern, according to the family, repeated itself nearly every day at dinnertime. The pattern was changed by a combination of experimentation with different eating techniques and the use of counseling techniques to help the family discover new ways to address the problem. It is not uncommon for speech-language-hearing problems to be embedded in family interactive patterns. In another case, a child with a language delay phonated; Mom imitated the vocalization; the child repeated the utterance; and both Mom and Dad cheered, smiled, patted the child, and showed pleasure in general. This was a pattern which we rewarded and, with the help of the parents, amplified. In a different family, a typical pattern was for Mom to say a word and then ask the child to say it. The child ignored Mom's repeated urgings, Dad showed annoyance with the child, Mom tried harder to encourage the child to say the word to no avail, and the child walked away. Mom then defended the child to Dad by saying something positive about him, and Dad responded with a look of disgust or displeasure. With both parent's help, this pattern was changed by finding a more effective way for Mom to encourage the child to speak. When the child responded appropriately, this successful interaction was discussed with Dad.

Fourth, *a family's structure, organization, and developmental stage are important factors in determining the behavior of family members* (Epstein & Bishop, 1981). Every family undergoes developmental changes over time, has a hierarchical structure, and adopts certain roles that are fulfilled by individual family members. Rules about the family's organization of these roles are often covert but are usually accepted and understood by each family member. For example, in a two-parent family with two young children and a grandmother living with the family (structure), the roles may be traditional in that the father is the primary breadwinner, the mother the primary caretaker, and the grandmother a respected but peripheral family member (roles). This family will organize itself around these roles with the parents assuming responsibility for managing the lives of the children (hierarchy). While the clinician may believe that the father should be more involved than he is, the right of the family to organize itself must be respected. It would be inappropriate, for example, to assign the uninvolved father to read stories to the communicatively disordered child. It would, however, be appropriate to honestly determine who usually would do such an activity and the circumstances under which it could be done and to enlist the father's support as the mother or grandmother carried out the task. As a family evolves over time, changes in society, family structure, and capabilities of the children will result in developmental changes necessitating different types of assignments.

Learning about how families organize themselves can be beneficial to the clinician who wishes to capitalize on this information in order to give meaningful assignments to family members. When a child is not talking, for example, the parents usually are aware of those techniques that are and are not successful in eliciting language. They know the child's reactions to different situations, when the time is appropriate to use an intervention, and when it is not. They also know the particular types of interactions with which each family member will be most successful. Further, while some families like to look at books, others like to play on the floor, or the mother likes to look at books with the children, but the father prefers active play. In some families, the father's role is to be supportive of the mother rather than to actually intervene in any active way. In other families, the grandmother may play an important role in child care, or stepparents may be actively involved with the child who has a communicative disorder.

As the clinician shows an understanding of the different family developmental stages, a respect for the family's structure, and an interest in the way the family assigns and organizes roles, she will be able to give assignments to family members that fit their individual strengths and styles.

FAMILY-BASED TREATMENT

Family-Based Treatment is a systemic, family-centered, solution-focused model for providing speech-language services in which counseling techniques are integrated into all aspects of the assessment and treatment process. The family, rather than the individual, is viewed as the unit of treatment; family members are involved in assessing their member's communicative strengths and weaknesses, discussing potential interventions, and using interventions in natural contexts to create positive communicative change in their member about whom they are concerned. The speech-language pathologist and family develop a partnership that increases in strength as services are provided

Unit of Treatment

When the individual is the unit of treatment, the context for assessment and rehabilitative services is the client-clinician dyad. The communicative disorder is understood and treated as it occurs in that setting. As such, the speech-language problem is viewed as a static condition of the individual even though the client may experience variations in different situations and the clinician understands that these may occur. The problem, however, is seldom actually seen by the clinician in other contexts for purposes of additional evaluation and treatment. Treatment is limited to time spent with the speech-language pathologist, and carryover of new behaviors into other situations is accepted as a potential problem.

When the family is the unit of treatment, the context for assessment, treatment, and change is the family-clinician system. Communication is evaluated and understood as it is manifested, shaped, and reacted to in the family. Treatment occurs in the natural, functional environment of the family, and carryover is not an issue since the clinician assists the family to effect change within real-life interactive situations. Family interactive patterns in which the communicative disorder is embedded may also be observed. This gives the clinician a greater depth of understanding of the problem and increases options for change.

Role of the Professional

In the individual model, treatment decisions are made by the professional and the client; family members are expected to comply with the habilitative plan. Consequently, when outside assignments are not completed, when the client arrives late for sessions, or the client appears disinterested, the client and/or family are said to be uncooperative.

In a Family-Based Treatment model the family becomes part of the solution and a member of the habilitative team. Family members participate in the assessment; have input as to the goals of treatment; and, with the help of the speech-language pathologist, utilize their resources to change the communicative behavior of their own family member. Compliance is not an issue when families participate at this level because each family's style of cooperating may be accessed and reinforced by the clinician.

Use of Counseling

Traditionally, information supplements the treatment process, and counseling is of an informative nature. The clinician attempts to help the client and/or family members understand what she is doing in treatment sessions and why this is important. The clinician typically uses professional language and attempts to teach the family to understand the problem in the same manner as it is understood by the clinician.

In a Family-Based Treatment model, counseling is integrated into the entire rehabilitative process. Counseling techniques are used by the clinician to promote family participation, to respond to attitudes and feelings that accompany disability, and to accomplish the tasks associated with each step of the process. The clinician builds upon the family's perspective of the problem to lead the family to a greater understanding of the communicative disorder and how it may be changed.

SUMMARY

Speech-language pathology services are steeped in the tradition of the individual medical model of service delivery. Efforts to include families and other professionals in clinical services have arisen out of assumptions associated with the traditional individual model. A systemic rather than a linear paradigm is necessary in order to effectively expand the influence of speech-language services through including families and others in treatment. The systemic model requires a shift in thinking about human behavior and an understanding of systems principles.

Family-Based Treatment is a systemic approach to clinical services in which families are involved in all aspects of assessment and treatment. The model offers both a theoretical framework and a process for providing services in the family context. An elaboration of many of the counseling techniques that are integrated with treatment will be discussed in Chapter 8.

CHAPTER 2

CONVENING THE FAMILY
AND
ESTABLISHING THE PARTNERSHIP

On rare occasions, family members will request permission to participate in treatment. In these cases the clinician begins family-centered treatment by arranging a convenient time and place for the first meeting. More often, family members are not accustomed to being included in the speech-language-hearing treatment process, and it is unlikely that they will request involvement. The clinician must take the initiative if family participation is desired.

ASSESSING THE PROFESSIONAL CONTEXT

Arranging a time when the family can meet with the clinician is the first, and sometimes most challenging, step in initiating family-centered services. The clinician must consider the opportunities and restrictions of his work setting. For example, some clinicians work in settings where parent conferences are an expected part of their services. These conferences may offer a natural opportunity to involve family members in a partnership relationship. Other clinicians may discover that family visits to long or short-term rehabilitation facilities offer an opportunity to talk with a key family member about convening significant others. Private practice or clinic settings offer clinicians the kind of flexibility that makes family-centered services an ideal treatment option. In other words, the clinician must evaluate possibilities for family involvement relative to the demands and expectations inherent in the professional context in which services will be offered.

Our work with families takes place in a university speech and hearing clinic, but the model is not limited to that context. Once a clinician decides to become systemic in his approach to treatment, and determines that this is possible in his clinical setting, the next step is to define the system and choose a convening strategy that will be successful.

DEFINING THE SYSTEM

Once the clinician has decided to integrate family involvement into his professional setting, he must decide whom to convene for the first meeting. We invite all of the family members who are significantly involved with the client. When the client is a child or adolescent living with both parents, we invite the parents as well as the child's siblings. All contribute to the environment in which the child lives, and all are affected and react to the client's situation. If the child lives with one parent and the other parent is nearby, we also invite the non-resident parent if the custodial parent is amenable to the idea. If the child's mother or father has remarried or is closely involved with another person, the step-parent or friend is also invited to the family meeting.

Sometimes grandparents, aunts, uncles, cousins, and/or close family friends have daily, significant contact with our clients. These people are invited to the first session if the adult in charge thinks that this is a good idea. More often, extended family members are not invited to first sessions but are included in future sessions. Extended family involvement, especially if there is frequent contact with the client, expands treatment options. We have been pleasantly surprised on several occasions to find grandparents, great-grandparents, aunts, cousins, playmates, baby-sitters and/or friends waiting with our families to join us in the treatment sessions. Family members seem to intuitively understand that these important people are significant members of the client's communicative environment.

When the client is an adult, with that person's agreement, we convene the spouse and any adult children who, with their spouses and children, are available to help in the treatment process. If the adult client lives alone or with one or both parents, the parents and/or available siblings are invited.

Occasionally the concept of family must be broadened to include foster parents, child care workers, residential facility counselors, inpatient treatment personnel or other professionals who interact on a daily basis with clients. The goal of convening is to invite family members and significant others based on their involvement with the client rather than beginning with a predetermined idea of a particular family organization. Families in our contemporary society are structured in a variety of ways, and the clinician must explore with the contact person all of the available options. The clinician should convene the people who are likely to expand an understanding of the interactive patterns in which the communicative disorder is embedded. All family members may not attend every session (if more than one meeting is desired), but when convened for the first meeting these people enrich the resource options available to the clinician and family.

CONVENING THE ENTIRE FAMILY

The Telephone Call

In our practice the initial family contact is made by telephone. Sometimes an introductory letter precedes the phone call or, as occasionally has been the case for us, the clients must be contacted by letter because they have no telephone. Some clinicians may have the opportunity to discuss a time and place to meet during family visits to a rehabilitation facility or when a parent stops by to pick up a child from a school facility. Often, however, telephone contact is the most efficient way to begin the convening process.

The joining process (see Chapter 8) begins with the first telephone or in-person contact. Information is exchanged and the partnership relationship is begun. For this reason we believe that the clinician, rather than an appointment secretary, should make the initial contact. Following is an example of a convening telephone call as it might occur in our practice:

Mother:	Hello.
Clinician:	Hello, this is Jim Andrews from the Speech & Hearing Clinic at Northern Illinois University. Donna Werner, the child development specialist, asked me to give you a call. She said you were interested in speech-language services for Nathan.
Mother:	Oh, yes, I am. I'm glad you called. We think he needs help with his speech; he's not talking much, and when he does talk, we can't understand him.
Clinician:	OK . . . we'll want to learn about that and figure out together what we can do to make some changes. I'll be mailing you a form to complete about your concerns. Who lives with you and Nathan?
Mother:	Well, his father who's at work right now . . . and his older sister, Missy . . she's six . . and his baby brother, Jake . . . he's 10 months.

Clinician: All right . . . the reason I'm asking is that when I'm working with a child, I like to have all of the family members participate. How does that sound to you?

Mother: OK, I guess. I don't know if my husband can come though. He usually works late and isn't too involved with things like this.

Clinician: He may not want to be real active in this, but I'd like to get both of your views of the situation and watch Nathan as he interacts with both of you. . . that's why we have evening hours, so that everyone can come.

Mother: OK, I think he'll come. But what about his sister and the baby? Do you want them to come too?

Clinician: Yes, them too. I especially like for everyone to be at the first session. Very young children don't have to come everytime, but I'd like to see how Nathan communicates with everyone. We see families at five, six, and seven o'clock on Mondays, Tuesdays, and Wednesdays. Sessions last no more than an hour . . . and we have an opening at 6:00 o'clock next Wednesday. Would that work for you?

Mother: Yes . . . I think so. Yes, six on Wednesday would be fine. That will give us time to eat something, and it still won't be too late for the kids.

Clinician: I know it's a real effort to bring the whole family, but we'll be working together, and I need your help so we can begin to make some changes. . . and, it's helpful to see how Nathan communicates with his sister and baby brother.

Mother: OK, actually, I kind of like the idea of bringing everyone because Missy, especially, is better at understanding Nathan than my husband and I are.

Clinician: That's often the case. Brothers and sisters can be very helpful.

Mother: I'll talk to John (husband) and make sure that 6:00 on Wednesday is all right with him. If there's a problem, I'll call you back; otherwise, we'll see you next Wednesday at 6:00.

Clinician: I'll mail you an assessment form to complete for our meeting on Wednesday, a parking card and a map. If for some reason you can't come, I'd appreciate a call.

Mother: OK. Is there anything we should do ahead of time?

Clinician: Yes, good idea. How about paying attention to the times that Nathan does use words, and notice what's going on when that happens.

Mother: OK, I'll try, and we'll all be there on Wednesday at 6:00 o'clock.

Clinician: OK, great . . . see you then.

Several issues are raised in this convening conversation. The first is the role of Nathan's father. Many fathers do not expect to be involved in treatment services, and most clinicians assume that the mother and child will be the treatment dyad if any family members participate. When the clinician adopts a systemic perspective, he knows that a clear understanding of family views and interactions will be elicited if, in a two-parent family, the father is included as well as the mother. Furthermore, the concerns that parents share when a child has special needs are more easily addressed when both parents are participants in the treatment process. Fathers are not always completely comfortable when they are first convened, but as their views are heard and respected, and as their resources are used, they usually enjoy participating in treatment. Children, also, seem to appreciate having both parents present. Siblings, of course, are also included and are excellent resources in many cases.

The second issue relates to the language used by the convening clinician. Notice the use of the phrase, "I need your help" and the related comments that imply that the family's help is needed. We have found this to be the single most useful phrase in our convening practice. We believe that family members have information to offer that will make our clinical work more successful. Eighteen years of working with families has not changed our perspective on this issue.

Third, the clinician acknowledged the hassle involved in gathering family members together. This conveys empathy for the sometimes overwhelming burdens that accompany issues of disability.

Finally, an intervention has already taken place – even before the meeting occurs. Since Nathan's mother asked for a task, she was given one that will provide a beginning focus for the first interview. A copy of the telephone intake form that we use is displayed in Appendix A, and the pre-assessment form we mail to families is displayed in Appendix B.

Each convening conversation is idiosyncratic to the clinician/client/family situation. The following issues should be kept in mind:

1. Begin with the goal of convening all of the members of the household that are an immediate part of the client's communicative context.

2. Use language of partnership and joining. Convey to family members at the outset that you know they will have valuable contributions to make to the treatment process.

3. Adopt an "experimental" attitude if you'd like. Tell family members that this is a new way of working for you – that it's a different way of treating speech-language problems, but exciting things can happen when clinicians work jointly with family members to help the client.

4. Be persistent. Your friendly insistence that you need the family members' ideas may not be fully heard at first. As you persist in letting the contact person know the importance of family participation, this desire will be heard and acknowledged. I (Jim) am unwilling to work with clients without family participation as I've learned that I'm a much more successful clinician with their help.

Scheduling

The desire to involve the members of the family may create complex scheduling issues. Some families can meet during regular daytime hours. Others can only meet after work and must be scheduled during the late afternoon and early evening. Some settings support flex-time arrangements, allowing the clinician to take morning time off in exchange for late afternoon availability. Flexibility in scheduling is critical to enlisting the cooperation of family members whose work hours vary.

However, the clinician must also assure that his own busy schedule is accommodated so that he does not resent giving up valuable personal time. It may be best to work with only one family if this is all that can reasonably be done. The clinician must feel energized and challenged by the exciting issues associated with family treatment, or the work will not be successful.

ESTABLISHING THE PARTNERSHIP

The speech-language pathologist or audiologist who genuinely believes that families have valuable resources for creating change and who encourages families to use these resources is likely to be successful in establishing successful partnerships with families. In Family-Based Treatment, the clinician seeks as many ways as possible to access the resources of the family as well as those of the client.

When the individual is the unit of treatment, it is customary to seek a level of rapport with the client. Probably everyone involved with students has seen lesson plans where the only goal was "to gain rapport" or its corollary, "to get to know the client." Most of us neither spend an hour on this goal alone nor assume that it can be completely accomplished in one session. We do, however, have a sense that it is important for clients to have a positive regard for us, and us for them, in order to gain their cooperation and thereby elicit change. It is no less important to seek a level of rapport with families when they are the unit of treatment. No one would show disrespect for a client or give the impression that he is not good enough to change, yet, inadvertently, this is the signal that families sometimes receive from members of helping professions. Under these circumstances, families may devalue their resources and lose confidence in their ability to participate effectively in services.

The following guidelines serve as reminders for us as much as for the reader. They were developed out of our experience in working with families and teaching the Family- Based Treatment model in classes and workshops. We use these reminders when convening families and throughout the treatment process

Respond to Family Members' Expertise

Families become active partners when they are acknowledged as experts about their own members and when their viewpoints are sought and appreciated. A family knows more about its member with a disability than anyone else. Combining the expertise of a family with that of the clinician can result in a powerful force for change. Families *assume* the expertise of the speech-language pathologist; that aspect of the relationship is a given. The speech-language pathologist, however, must overtly acknowledge the expertise of families and assure them that the information they offer is valuable. Since this acknowledgment is not necessarily part of the typical family-professional relationship, family members may need to be convinced that their expertise is desired.

Acknowledge Family Members' Emotions

Families cooperate most when they are allowed to express emotions and feelings about their family members in an empathic atmosphere. Not all professionals are comfortable in the presence of a client or family member who is discouraged, crying, or angry. It is not difficult to show in many nonverbal ways, as well as through verbal responses, that emotions of distress are not welcome. This may even be the most efficient way to conduct individual treatment sessions. When family members are involved, however, strong emotions are likely to be expressed from time to time. Responses from the clinician that are most helpful are those that restate or reflect the feelings being expressed. These skills are discussed in Chapter 8. Responses that are least helpful are those that give advice, attempt to encourage the person or to cheer him/her up, minimize the problem, change the subject, or seek more facts. In many cases, after expressing emotions in an atmosphere of acceptance and understanding, the family shows renewed energy and an increased appreciation for the family-clinician relationship.

Respect Family Members' Concerns

Families cooperate most when their very strong concerns about their member who is disabled are viewed objectively and empathically. Many of the families with whom we work have sought services which seemed unnecessary or even useless to us. Angela, a three-year-old with mental retardation, was treated by a chiropractor in hopes that spinal adjustments would help her. Gina, age six with autistic-like behavior, began a program of patterned limb motion and eye exercises because her parents thought it might improve her behavior. Tom, fifteen years old and cerebral palsied, had his tongue clipped and underwent massive orthodontia in hopes that his tongue would move better if it had more room. These are just a few examples of the efforts of families to help their children. In no case was our opinion sought. These families wanted to help their children, not discuss rationales or hear professional disagreements. If our opinion had been asked, we would have given it. Since it was not, we attempted to join the families in their concern for the family member and desire to do everything possible. Responding to the emotions that led to their decision, joining them in their desire for change, using neutral questions (see Chapter 8) to learn more about the supplementary services, and using the services in a positive way all seemed more likely to be effective than showing skepticism or questioning the family's judgment.

Allow Family Imperfection

Families cooperate most when the clinician recognizes and encourages their ability to change and accepts that families and, indeed, clinicians will not do everything perfectly. Most of us have learned that treatment is most effective when we do everything perfectly. This occurs when the reinforcement schedule is exactly right, when we provide models and fade them at just the right time, when we choose stimuli for practice that contain only selected phonemic sequences, etc. We are not disappointed when change does not follow immediately; rather, we keep experimenting with our interventions and responses to the client. Further, we think of a sequence of treatment; no one expects the problem to be corrected in one session. When working with families, it seems easy to forget this. Rather than viewing efforts to identify and use family resources over time, it is easy to become impatient and think of the family as being difficult rather than examining our own interventions and responses to families and viewing family participation as a process.

Families will not do everything perfectly in the beginning, if ever. However, by combining our expertise with theirs, we believe that our services often can be substantially more effective than if we worked alone with the client. Even if we *could* do treatment perfectly (and most of us can't), enlisting the family augments all treatment goals.

Appreciate Interactive Uniqueness

Families cooperate most when the clinician tries to understand the problem as it occurs in the interactive context of each family. Communicative disorders manifest themselves in different ways in different settings. For example, a child with a language delay is likely to use more words at home with his family than at a preschool or in the presence of the clinician when the attention of everyone in the room is on the child. If families are to make interventions in the environment of the home, it is important that clinicians understand the manner in which family members experience the problem. As we begin to understand the problem within the context of the family, then we may make valid and useful suggestions for them to carry out and build upon between sessions.

Create Idiosyncratic Assignments

Families cooperate most when the clinician understands each speech-language problem from the family's perspective and uses this information to give appropriate assignments that fit the family's understanding of the problem. Family members must understand the purpose and desired outcome of each assignment, or they will be unable to accommodate to variations in the behavior and responses of their family member with a communicative disorder. When including families, it may be a greater priority for the clinician to understand the problem from the point of view of the family than for the family to understand the problem from the clinician's perspective; both, however, are important.

Enable Family Members

Family members cooperate most when the clinician is genuinely willing to enable them to recognize their rightful role to make decisions about their own member's treatment and to experience the satisfaction of improvement. When we work with individuals, we are accustomed to receiving a measure of credit for the change that we presumably evoked. When families are participants in treatment, the credit for change is shared with family members. In some cases, families may even attribute the change to a third factor or indicate that they do not know why the problem no longer exists.

Robert's parents, for example, attributed the fact that he no longer stuttered to their reducing the amount of sugar he was allowed to add to his breakfast cereal. This change was made along with rather far-reaching changes in their family interactive patterns, particularly with Robert. While our view of the relative importance of these two "causes" of change was different from that of the family's, the family made *both* changes. The important point is to reward parents for their involvement and empower them to continue to influence behavior rather than to quibble over reasons for change.

SUMMARY

Upon deciding to take a systemic approach and include families in the treatment process, the next task is to determine how to convene the family. The initial contact will be successful if the clinician uses language that signals participation and non-judgmental acceptance. All family members should be present for the clinician to view the family interactions in which the disorder is embedded. A certain amount of friendly persistence may be necessary to achieve the goal of all family members being present, particularly fathers who are not accustomed to being invited. Flexibility in scheduling is necessary, but the clinician must arrange his time so that working with families is an exciting and challenging process. Family members will join the clinician in an effective partnership when the clinician responds to their expertise, acknowledges their emotions, respects their concerns, allows imperfection, appreciates interactive uniqueness, creates idiosyncratic assignments, and enables family members to recognize their right to empowerment.

CHAPTER 3

SHARING AN UNDERSTANDING OF THE PROBLEM

There are many different ways of thinking about and understanding communicative disorders. Just as the clinician shares a view of the problem when offering services based on the individual direct services model, it is important when working systemically, for the clinician to develop and share a clear view of the problem. In many cases that view will be the one adopted by the family. On the other hand, unlike the individual model of services in which the different views held by family members may be irrelevant, when family members are participants in treatment, it is important for the clinician to understand their perspectives of the problem.

The process in which each member of the family describes how the problem is experienced and understood is itself an intervention. That process usually leads the family to a greater understanding of the communicative disorder, the ways that family members have reacted to it, and interventions that each person has attempted. In turn, by learning this information, the clinician is in a better position to understand solutions offered by the family. The clinician can then describe her own view of the problem in a way that is meaningful to the family and suggest solutions that accommodate the family's perspective.

When solutions suggested by the clinician are framed in language that fits the family's explanation and understanding of the problem, the suggestions may be said to be isomorphic to the family's view. Isomorphism is defined by Hofstadter (1979) as a situation in which "two complex structures can be mapped onto each other, in such a way that to each part of one structure there is a corresponding part in the other structure" (p. 49). It is a family therapy principle that isomorphic assignments are more likely to be followed by families than assignments that do not relate to the family's understanding of the problem (deShazer, 1982). In other words, when the clinician understands the manner in which family members view the problem, she is

31

in a position to offer more effective suggestions for change than if the family's views remain unknown. This and other features of assignments will be discussed in Chapter 5.

Since most speech-language pathologists employ a direct services model of clinical practice, traditionally we have assumed that the clinician should learn about the problem in order to personally treat it. On the other hand, when adopting a systemic perspective, the clinician's goal is to learn about the problem in a way that will permit everyone within the defined system to participate in treating it. This difference is substantial and affects all phases of the assessment process.

A number of counseling techniques may be used when interacting with family members. These enable the clinician to gain admittance to the family system, learn about the problem from the family, respond to their concerns, and enlist family members' participation in treatment. These counseling techniques are mentioned in conjunction with the process step of sharing an understanding of the problem described in this chapter, but will be discussed in Chapter 8. They include joining, clarifying, reflecting, summarizing, tracking interactive patterns, neutral questioning, and creative strategizing.

USING A POLYOCULAR PERSPECTIVE TO LEARN THE FAMILY'S VIEW

At the outset, we anticipate that each family member will view the potential speech-language problem slightly differently. We particularly want to probe for varying perspectives since they may introduce "news of difference" (Bateson, 1979) and suggest idiosyncratic treatment options, as previously discussed. These emerge as each person describes his perspective, later in the session after the process of establishing a partnership has begun.

Once the family is convened, it is useful to begin the meeting with a few joining remarks. Reiterating that family members' willingness to participate is appreciated and explaining, again, why the entire family is involved is usually helpful since it is different than what they might have expected. Reminding the family that they are experts about their member, that they know more about their family member than anyone else, and that their help is needed to solve the problem assures them that they will be an integral part of the treatment team.

If children are involved, it is helpful for parents to know the ground rules. When toys are set out, the clinician may indicate that, if the parents wish, it is all right for the children to play with them. If there are objects that children should not disturb, this too should be indicated to the parents. This affirms at the outset the appropriate role of parents and indicates to them that they will be in charge of their children. The clinician may ask the family to bring a few toys and/or books that their child enjoys. This provides an even greater opportunity to learn about the family since it increases their control over the situation and tends to evoke their typical interactive style.

Very early it is likely that the clinician will notice behaviors and interactions that seem to be potential resources for intervention. These should be remembered for future use. It is not, however, inappropriate to comment upon something that a family member does that is exceptionally useful. When a family member interacts with the client in such a way that the client responds with behavior that is obviously desirable, the clinician may speak positively of the intervention by talking about how well or how appropriately the client responded to that family member.

After addressing or attending to each family member, it is time to learn about the problem in a more formal manner. The clinician can begin this phase with a general statement such as, "Tell us about Andy" or "Let's talk about what you've noticed as you interact with Andy." It may be a small point, but this type of statement indicates that there's more to Andy than a "problem," and it encourages families to think about Andy as a person, even in a situation in which attention eventually will be focused upon his communicative ability. The family spokesperson usually responds first. After the family spokesperson has described the communicative problem from her perspective, a convenient method for making the transition to other family members is to say something like, "What do you think about that, Mr. Davis? What have you noticed?" Children should also be offered the opportunity to respond if they have been listening to the conversation. The question to children may be addressed in the form of whether or not the brother or sister with the communicative disorder talks to them or whether or not they can understand their sibling. A request for a brief description of how the children play together or, what each sibling does when the brother or sister cannot be understood may be made. If the children have been playing together as the adults conversed, comments may be made about the manner in which siblings interacted with the child about whom the family is concerned. We often see older siblings attempting to help their younger brother or sister who is not as adept at communicating as they are. This is consistent, of course, with the systemic principle that everyone is affected by the speech-language impairment and that everyone reacts to it and attempts to help the person.

When the client is an adolescent or adult, the same process is followed, but more attention is given to that person's view of the problem than is usually the case with young children. As the adolescent or adult expresses his/her views, the clinician must be careful to attend in a way that respects and acknowledges the client's hierarchical position in the family. As a general rule, attention to the views of the client increases with the individual's age until adulthood is reached.

Identifying Interactive Patterns

As family members are describing the problem, the clinician should attend to descriptions of interactive patterns related to the communicative disorder. Tracking interactive sequences is a counseling technique that is used to learn about patterns in which the communicative problem is embedded. This technique leads to detailed descriptions of family interactions. Descriptive sequences of who says what and when can be developed, much like the script of a play. Each sequence in the script usually begins either with the client attempting to communicate or with a family member attempting to elicit responses or communication from the client. From that point on, the clinician may ask about each behavioral event in the communicative sequence. We suggest listening, particularly, for successful interactions (eg., where a parent helped the child, the child said the word, the intent of the child was understood, etc.) but also for those interactions that ended in frustration. Leading families to describe their communicative attempts at home and encouraging them to think about things they already have done to help their family member, not only gives the clinician information, but it usually results in families arriving at a new level of understanding of their situation. New insights grow out of the experience of describing events that occur at home. It is most important at this time not to give advice, but rather to listen and to use tracking and other techniques in order to gain a clear understanding of the problem as it occurs in the family environment.

Interactive sequences also are likely to be acted out by family members during this first and subsequent sessions. As stated earlier, it is not too early for the clinician to compliment parents or other family members for those things that they say or do that appear to be helpful and that may facilitate change. We believe that it is far more useful to reinforce helpful things that family members say and do than to point out interactions that seem inappropriate. The latter are remembered, however, and discussed at later sessions if they continue to perpetuate the problem in a significant way.

It is particularly important, but sometimes difficult, to allow the family to show its interactive style. It is impossible to give meaningful assignments to families without knowing something about the environment in which they will be carried out. Allowing the family to "show itself" may at first seem like wasting time or losing control since, traditionally, we are accustomed to structuring the environment and reducing distractions to a minimum. However, a clinician gains insights and understands the problem more completely by observing and experiencing the environment in which the communicative disorder is manifested on an everyday basis. Further, the clinician is likely to personally sense the same feelings as the family as she joins the family system. We continue to be surprised by the power and ability of families to transmit to us their tension, frustration, sense of hopelessness, happiness, and other emotions.

Identifying Mobilization Points

If family members do not volunteer what they do to help their family member, we always ask. We have never worked with a family that had not already attempted to help their child or other member with a speech-language problem. We believe that this is an inevitable natural reaction with much potential for clinicians. We listen for successful techniques to build upon and for unsuccessful techniques to avoid. From the family's point of view, those strategies that seem to be successful, already make sense to them. These will be easier for them to expand upon than new techniques which they have never used or experienced. We think of these successful, natural interactive techniques as mobilization points (Scott, 1984). They are one part of the family's resources and are excellent points from which to begin treatment.

It is also useful to learn about typical family activities in which the client is involved, especially everyday events and times when one or more family members interact with the individual. These provide opportunities for family members to intervene. Learning about the client's favorite activities and typical daily events often suggests related opportunities for functional interventions by persons in the environment.

Listening for Agreement/Disagreement

During this initial portion of the interview and throughout the treatment process, it is important to listen for and talk about disagreements expressed between family members. The most common disagreement we have experienced is that one parent is more concerned about the perceived problem than the other. When this is the case, and after talking openly about the two different views, we typically summarize the two perspectives and try to find a point of accommodation: "Mr. Jones, it sounds like you aren't really too concerned because you were also late in talking, and Kathy may outgrow this just like you did. But, Mrs. Jones, you're pretty worried about

Kathy and would like to do something about it right now. Mr. Jones, would you be willing to participate in services to help ease your wife's concern?" In essentially every case in which this particular situation has come up, the answer to our question has been a genuine "yes." This intervention frees both parents to later observe and listen to the speech-language pathologist in a different way than if the issue had never been resolved. Both family members in this example become joined with one another and with the clinician in the effort to determine an appropriate level of service.

We believe that disagreements that are ignored will return to impede progress. It is very important, then, to listen carefully for these, talk about them, and try to find a point of accommodation. This is not to imply that family members all experience the communicative disorder in the same way or that each should think about it like everyone else in the family. These disagreements should be highlighted, but no point of agreement will be sought. Rather, the clinician will determine interventions that take advantage of the different experiences and perspectives. It is helpful to talk about differences positively. For example, "Brian is lucky to have both of your influences. Dad, you like to roughhouse with him and don't worry about how much he talks; on the other hand, Mom, you're concerned about how he'll fit into school next year, and you like to stimulate him academically. Both of these are important." Assignments that follow should capitalize on the two different parental styles.

A frequent question that arises is whether the person with the communicative disorder should be present during this portion of the interview. Without that individual present, it is impossible to assess his/her role as a communicator in the family system, the manner in which family members interact with that person, and the communicative environment of the family. These interactions are so important that they should be observed even if detailed questions about the individual with the handicap are not asked in his/her presence. In all but a very small number of cases, we have included the family member with the problem in the room with everyone else. That person nearly always knows that he/she is the reason for the conference. Further, the conversation about the problem is conducted in a caring manner. This may be quite different from the manner in which the problem has been discussed at home and also different from the giving of advice or cajoling that may have occurred in other contexts. On the other hand, if it seems inappropriate to talk about the problem in the client's presence, don't do it. A clinician's judgment should never be superseded by the dictates of a particular approach.

DEVELOPING THE CLINICIAN'S VIEW

After learning about the problem from the family's perspective, observing interactions in which the problem is embedded, and observing the manner in which the client communicates, a more detailed assessment is necessary. At this point, the clinician needs to learn more about the problem and determine additional information about possibilities for change. Since the bulk of change is likely to occur in interactions with family members, it is important to include them as active participants in the assessment. This not only leads to further information about the communicative disorder but allows the clinician to determine the nature of family resources that are available.

Family Participation

The specific manner in which the family participates in the assessment varies with the type of communicative disorder. A primary goal, however, is to include family members in such a way that they appreciate the problem more completely and see themselves as capable of eliciting change in their own family member. The latter is a source of empowerment for families. It usually is rewarding to families to be able to change even a small aspect of their family member's communicative ability very early in the treatment process. Initial suggestions should take this into account and be directed toward a behavior that is amenable to change.

The clinician may begin by attending to that part of the problem that concerns family members most. For example, when the primary concern is articulation, administration of an articulation test can yield useful information about family resources for participating in treatment. The clinician can start by briefly explaining the nature of the test and asking a family member to administer it. Seating is rearranged to allow family members and the clinician to sit close to the child. Initially, as each picture is named, the clinician may comment on the child's accuracy of production usually adding a brief statement about how the particular sound is produced. When a sound is misarticulated, the clinician provides a model for the child and elicits imitation. Appropriate feedback is given to the child by the clinician. Family members observe these interactions and after the clinician has done this two or three times, the member administering the test is asked to do the stimulability testing/trial therapy. From that point, the clinician should attend to both the parent and the child and comment upon the performance of each. Just as verbal directions and reinforcement are traditionally used to shape the behavior of clients, the same techniques are used with the family member. The reactions of other family members are also observed and the ability of the parent administering the test is positively described to them. It is particularly useful to comment on the helpful techniques that the family member is using. For example, "You let him know really well that you were pleased when he corrected the way he made that sound" or "I like the way you're exaggerating the sound to help her; that calls it to her attention." Just as we want individual clients to feel good about their ability to change, we want parents and other family members to have that same sense of satisfaction. The clinician may then reinforce both the parent and the child, but gradually the role of reinforcing the child is turned over to the parent. The clinician is commenting throughout on the child's speech, teaching the family as the clinician learns. The clinician may also compare performance on the test to spontaneous speech as heard earlier by the clinician or commented upon by family members.

When the problem is language delay with a young child, the clinician can begin the clinical assessment by asking an appropriate family member to play with the child for a few minutes. During this time, the clinician may observe features such as ability to obtain a shared focus of attention with the child; the extent to which the parent follows the child's lead, provides models, and otherwise stimulates the child; the frequency with which the parent reinforces desired behavior, etc. Both the child's responses and the adult's style of interaction are observed and mentally compared with earlier descriptions and observations. Gradually, the clinician inserts himself/herself into the activity. Often the first step is to comment on either something the parent is doing well or to join the parent in his/her frustration by commenting upon something that is difficult (eg., getting the child's attention). Rather than "taking over," the clinician should *join* the parent(s) and child in play. While interacting with the child, the clinician can comment on the child's responses to interventions and the child's playing style. This interaction permits the clinician to determine the client's responses to different forms of stimulation and reward and to gain a sense of those behaviors that will be easiest to change. Gradually, the clinician may use different techniques to elicit words or model a style of interaction that appears to the clinician to be useful. He may also suggest a new activity to experiment further if the parents or the child do not change activities on their own.

When the client is older, the interactive context for this portion of the evaluation is usually more conversational. For example, the family with a family member who has aphasia or a head injury may be asked to engage in conversation to demonstrate some of the features that they described earlier during the interview. In this case the clinician observes the interactions and may begin to make comments, particularly noting helpful interventions made by family members. In some cases, of course, these involve a passive behavior such as waiting; whereas in others, the interaction may be more active, such as saying the first sound of a word. We especially want to notice the reaction of the client to these attempts to help. If the intervention made communication easier, this should be confirmed with the client, if possible, and with the family members. Such behavior may be a mobilization point. If the client appeared to become angry or frustrated by the intervention, this too should be discussed. These brief discussions often lead to descriptions of related attempts to help and the effectiveness of these efforts. These, too, may be demonstrated by the family during the session.

Gradually, the clinician becomes part of the conversation and makes his/her own interventions. Since these are done with the family present as participants, they will observe the effectiveness of the clinician's suggestions and comment upon how they relate to techniques they have tried. In the case of a head-injured mildly apraxic teenager, for example, we suggested that he emphasize the rhythm of his speech. At the first session we selected phrases we heard him use spontaneously in interactions with his parents and siblings. By having him practice these, we were able to develop an assignment at the first meeting that everyone understood. Since the young man enjoyed playing the drums, his mother suggested that he tap out the rhythm of selected words, phrases, and sentences on his leg. His older brother suggested phrases that the client tended to use in conversation while his father told us the words that were especially difficult for his son to say. The teenager also contributed to this discussion and made suggestions. Through the combined efforts of the clinician and the family, an evaluation of functional communication took place, goals were set, and an assignment for the first week was developed.

Standardized Testing

When using a systemic approach, the clinician may increasingly evaluate communication in functional contexts and rely less and less on standardized tests. While the former leads directly to interventions (as described above), the latter usually does not. When a standardized test is administered, however, one can begin by explaining the purpose and nature of the test. The clinician can explain that the client may not respond to some items that family members are sure he/she knows. Other responses, however, may be pleasantly surprising to the family. The clinician should make it clear that the test must be administered in a particular manner. The family may be advised that the group will discuss the client's performance after the test is completed. Further, the clinician may add that she realizes that it is sometimes difficult to watch quietly as a test is administered. Nevertheless, the family should watch. However, if the family includes small children who may distract the client it is appropriate to have someone take the children to another room while the test is being administered. After completing the test, families usually want to talk about their observations and compare them with their everyday experience. Sometimes, as a result of watching, families will come to a new realization of the seriousness and severity of the problem. In this case, the clinician can follow the family's lead and discuss the problem in more detail. Counseling skills are used to respond to emotional statements and behavior. When families are expressing their concern and/or grief XE "grief", it is no time for advice, suggestions, cheering up, or minimizing the problem. The most helpful thing that the clinician can do at that time is to respond to the feelings being expressed.

SUMMARY

In the first phase of the assessment, we are suggesting that the clinician learn each family member's view of the problem and listen particularly for (1) interactive sequences in which the problem is embedded; (2) mobilization points; (3) times when family members come together with the communicatively handicapped member; (4) activities which both the handicapped member and other family members enjoy doing together; and (5) agreement/disagreement between family members. This information may be enhanced by observing interactions as they are acted out during the session.

After learning about the family's view of the problem, the clinical evaluation is performed with family participation. It is suggested that the clinician talk about what she is learning throughout this portion of the assessment so that by the time it is completed, the family will have learned about the problem along with the clinician. This allows the family to participate more effectively in treatment than if the clinician were to conduct the evaluation privately.

CHAPTER 4

AGREEING ON CHANGES AND SETTING GOALS

Both the speech-language pathologist and the family will be burgeoning with new information after sharing an understanding of the problem. For the family, the process has involved hearing one another's view of their situation, often for the first time. They will have discovered points of agreement and disagreement and outlined the specifics of their interactions with the family member having a communicative disorder. Having heard one another describe what each person has done to help, the family is likely to be thinking about the problem and potential solutions in a new way. The speech-language pathologist's professional energy has been focused on learning about the problem from the different family members including the family member with the communicative disorder. The clinician has observed enactments of interactive patterns, conducted a clinical assessment, and developed a view of the problem. Finally, the clinician has been thinking about how his professional knowledge can be linked to the family's resources. Both family members and the clinician have a developing sense of the problem and of the early possibilities for change. Successful family participation now depends upon the clinician's expertise in applying his knowledge in a manner that will be useful to the family. The skill required is quite different than that which would be used in a direct service delivery model. It is natural to have reservations about one's ability to do this; sometimes mistakes will be made just as errors are made in individual treatment sessions. The difference, however, is that no one knows about mistakes of judgment made in a closed client-clinician dyad. Working with families requires both confidence in one's clinical ability and an open style of interacting.

When the first goal of treatment is not obvious and clear to everyone, the clinician can begin the goal-setting phase of services by asking the family to suggest one or two behaviors in which even a small change would be significant to them. If their request is not inconsistent with the principles of good speech-language pathology practice, it should be honored. In fact, rather than refusing an inappropriate request, the clinician can suggest modifications to make the request an appropriate goal.

Recently, along with our students, we have been experimenting with the use of a scaling procedure that supports the setting of both short-term and long-term goals by family members. We have used this technique with families having young children, but it can also be used with adults who are setting goals for themselves. Scaling is a strategy described and used by solution-focused psychotherapists (Berg, 1994; Butler & Powers, 1996; De Jong & Berg, 1998; deShazer, 1988; O'Hanlon & Weiner-Davis, 1989; Selekman, 1993; Walter & Peller, 1992). The basic procedure is to rate the client's communicative skill on a ten-point scale. A rating of "1," we explain to parents, describes the child's communication at the time the speech-language appointment was made and "10" is consistent with the child communicating at an excellent level. "Where," we ask, "would you place your child's communication on that one to ten scale right now?" Once parents have made their choices, the clinician engages the family in a discussion of the characteristics of the child's present communicative efforts. The clinician summarizes this information and re-states that this behavior is represented by the number each person has assigned. We then ask the family what they think the child will be doing when they believe he is showing significantly improved communication and to give that a number. We often add that at that level they may feel that speech-language services are no longer needed. They proceed to describe that behavior and assign a number, typically between 7 and 9. The speech-language characteristics they describe for that rating become the long-term goal of treatment.

Once the child's present level is scaled and described, and the long-term goals have been set, the next step is to determine what the child would be doing if his communication were to be rated one-half to one point higher. In other words, "Right now, you rated Joey's communication at about a 4. What would it take to bring him up to 4 1/2 or 5? What would he be doing if he were communicating at that level?" The purpose of this question is to assist family members in setting a short-term goal and to encourage them to begin thinking about change occurring in "small steps." The question usually engenders additional discussion among family members, and finally each person describes the new behavior. This communicative behavior becomes the short-term goal. The clinician then searches for exceptions: "Are there *any* times when Joey shows that behavior or something approaching it *now*?" Typically, family members are able to describe one or more situations when the new behavior, or something approximating it, has occurred. The details of that situation are discussed, and the clinician uses amplification to suggest that one or more family members have done something to facilitate that behavior. This leads to suggestions that become the assignment (see Chapter 5).

Scaling is a flexible technique that may be used in various ways by the clinician. Sometimes, we ask family members to rate their family member's communication at the time the appointment was made and we mentally compare that rating with the rating given at the time of the first or second session. This use of the technique may be used to explore pre-treatment changes, i.e., change that has occurred since making the initial appointment for assessment and treatment. Sometimes we describe the range (1 to 10) and set 10, ourselves, as the rating that would be given when the family believes that treatment is no longer necessary. Other times we ask family members to ascribe a number at which they would believe that their family member would no longer need speech-language services. In either case, we ask family members to describe the associated behavior their family member would be showing. An example of the way we used scaling with one of our families is given in Chapter 9.

When scaling is not used, family members typically prefer that the professional decide what the goals should be. By this time in the process, families have been involved in a mutual sharing of ideas and information and understand that they will be active participants in making changes. As respect is shown for the family they, in turn, become respectful of the opinions of the speech-language pathologist in a manner characteristic of "equal partners." Even when the clinician sets the treatment goals, he can offer the family an opportunity to confirm or ratify the decision. This is an important step since it is critical that family members understand and agree to the specifics of the particular behavior to be changed. The point is that family members, client and clinician together decide on treatment goals based upon mutually derived understandings.

Resources of the family, including mobilization points, form a major basis for setting goals and determining behaviors to be changed. The process of family participation in changing the behavior of one of its members early in treatment is probably as important as the details of the behavior selected and the magnitude of change relative to the overall problem. Just as we design goals and procedures in a direct services model so that the individual will be highly successful, in a systemic model the clinician will want to arrange success for both the client and the family members participating in treatment.

The clinician's internal process of connecting his expertise with the family's idiosyncratic style is called *creative strategizing* (see Chapter 8). The clinician attempts to combine all of the information he has learned about the family's view of the problem, the family's style and structure, scaling responses, mobilization points, and the clinician's own view of what can and should be changed in order to develop appropriate goals and related assignments. This process is repeated at subsequent sessions, but additional information is added based upon the outcome of assignments.

Four examples of first session information follow. The initial goal(s) and assignments that were developed with these families are also described. These case studies serve to describe the process more than to exemplify perfection!

FAMILY NUMBER ONE

Present at the first session: Kate, 4 years, 2 months; mother, Mildred (divorced); live-in boy friend, Jerry; and, eight-year-old brother, Greg.
Chief Complaint: Difficulty understanding Kate's speech
Family Characteristics and Interactions:
1. Kate talks > mother can't understand what Kate says > mother asks Kate to repeat what she said > (a) Kate speaks more clearly > (mother rewards Kate, sometimes) > mother responds, or (b) mother still can't understand Kate and tells Kate this > Kate walks away.
2. Kate has opportunities to talk; family members wait for her and try to understand what she says.
3. Mother and friend are capably in charge of the children and have established a calm, pleasant environment.

Mobilization Points:
1. Mother reinforces Kate, and Kate responds well to her praise.
2. Mother's friend enjoys singing songs, reading books to the children, and making up stories with the children.
3. Kate corrects many of her error sounds with minimal stimulation.

Speech-Language Characteristics:
1. Simplification of blends
2. t/k prevocalically
3. w/l or /l/ omitted
4. Inconsistent errors on multisyllabic words with moderate difficulty sequencing syllables
5. Inconsistent use of /f/ for plosives and fricatives; most common in blends (eg., tr > fr; gr > fr; dr > fr; gl > fr; br > fr; kr > fr)
6. Inconsistent use of me/I

Initial Goals:
1. Correct use of /k/ in prevocalic position
2. Improve ability to sequence sounds and syllables accurately by attending to the rhythm of speech

First Assignment:
1. Make a list of songs you like to sing with Kate and bring it next week. When you sing with her this week, listen especially for three syllable words in the songs and notice how they sound.
2. Find excuses for Kate to hear you say a lot of words that start with the "k" sound (eg., when playing, singing, telling stories, etc.). Emphasize them a little by pausing briefly and saying them with a little more force than usual.

After discussing the assignment with the family and demonstrating the technique, the family spontaneously named some words beginning with the /k/ sound that came up frequently in conversations with Kate. These were the following: comb, car, Kate, come, curtain, and kitchen. A session was scheduled for the next week.

In a one-hour session, a good deal was learned about Kate's speech and how her family could help her. More information would be developed in the continuing weeks, but enough was learned at the first session to establish initial goals and procedures to elicit change. The resources of the mother became especially apparent when she participated in administering an articulation test. She learned immediately how to stimulate and reward Kate in a kind, patient, natural manner. Kate's brother helped us learn about Jerry's story-telling assets and enjoyment of play when we asked about times that the family enjoyed being together. It was clear from the beginning that the adults were in charge of the children and that family members' rights were important and protected. As we joined the family system, we sensed a combination of respect, enjoyment, and playfulness.

The goals were selected by us, but the family was given the opportunity to agree or disagree with them. The /k/ was selected as a target sound since Kate used it correctly in many phonetic contexts, and her mother was able to stimulate a correct production rather easily. Further, both adults were able to identify it and easily distinguish it from /t/. Note, however, that their initial assignment was not to correct Kate's production but, rather to let her hear the sound. Interestingly, while playing alone at the next session, Kate used the sound correctly in words she said aloud as the adults were discussing the success of the assignment. Emphasizing Kate's use of rhythm, we believed, would provide a framework for the general improvement of articulation. This goal was particularly directed toward improving her inconsistent sequential errors in multisyllabic words. The family's enjoyment of singing songs with Kate provided a vehicle for a beginning emphasis upon the rhythm of speech.

During the first session, the family's resources were called to their attention prior to giving the assignment. Reinforcing a family's resources has the effect of enlisting their cooperation and strengthening family members' abilities and confidence to change their own member's behavior. Setting goals and determining methods for changing behavior so that these may be utilized has the effect of enabling families to participate effectively.

FAMILY NUMBER TWO

Present at the first session: Steve, 16 years (head injured); mother, Margaret; father, John; sister, Karen, 19 years; brother, Ed, 14 years.
Chief Complaint: Slurred hesitant speech and difficulty finding words following the head trauma.
Family Characteristics and Interactions:
1. The family is appropriately attentive to Steve and wants to help him. Their main concern had been his health and survival, but they are now eager to normalize his life.
2. Steve's mother and sister do most of the talking for the family, but defer appropriately to Steve and allow him to speak for himself.
3. Steve is given time to think of words and has ample opportunities to participate in conversation

Mobilization Points:
1. Steve has figured out that his speech is best when he speaks slowly and deliberately. He tries to help himself in this way.
2. Steve's parents have encouraged his musical and theatrical interests through private lessons in both areas. Further, he has been active in athletics and is a successful student.
3. The entire family is interested in music; all play musical instruments and some are members of orchestras.
4. Steve and his family brought a list of words that were particularly difficult for him to say.

Speech-Language Characteristics:
  1. Mild verbal apraxia
  2. Mild word finding problem
  3. Sentence formulation and grammatical structure were very good.
  4. Speech less animated, less colloquial, and more monotonous in pitch and loudness than prior to the injury. Steve's friends described him as "more formal" and "not as fun loving" as previously.
  5. Very mild dysarthria associated with weakness on the right side of the lips and tongue. Tongue deviated to the right upon protrusion. No apparent atrophy or fasciculations.
  6. Immediate memory mildly impaired.

Initial Goal:
  To reduce the apraxic-related errors in conversation

First Assignment:
  1. Experiment with directing speech movements with your head or tapping with your hand to exaggerate and get a sense of the rhythm of speech.
  2. Have "think rhythm" conversations with family members in which you exaggerate the rhythm of speech for a minute or two.
  3. Practice the seven words that you brought which are especially difficult for you in the phrases below. Exaggerate the rhythm of the phrases.
                I'm going to be <u>practicing</u>.
                Tomorrow is <u>Thursday</u>.
                It's got the <u>same sound</u>.
                Don't be <u>gullible</u>.
                Don't be <u>facetious</u>.
                DeKalb, <u>Illinois</u>
                Topics of <u>conversation</u>

The initial goal was related to one of the concerns expressed by Steve and his family. The intervention procedures grew out of a combination of Steve's discovery that he could improve his articulation if he spoke more deliberately, the clinician's knowledge of the nature of apraxia, and practice during the session in which Steve's articulation improved greatly when he exaggerated the rhythm of speech. His ability to sense the rhythm of speech was connected to the family's musical ability and interests and Steve's excellent pre-injury drum playing ability. This prompted the family to experiment with Steve in a different manner than if that association had not been made.

Steve was reinforced for his introspective ability to figure out that there were things he could do to help himself. The family's obvious concern for Steve and their desire to restore normalcy to his life were positively regarded by the clinician. Subsequent assignments capitalized on his voice lessons, acting interest, drumming ability, his pre-injury sense of humor, and his desire to succeed academically. The latter two became mobilization points as both behaviors began to improve.

FAMILY NUMBER THREE

Present at the first session: Sam, 3 years, 10 months; mother, Lana; father, Gene; brother, Tom, 18 months.

Chief Complaint: Parents can't understand Sam's speech.

Family Characteristics and Interactions:

1. Sam's mother is the family spokesperson and is worried about Sam's communicative performance. Sam's father is quiet, not very worried about Sam, but supportive of his wife.

2. Much of the family's interaction focuses upon or relates to Sam. Interactions are designed to promote his communicative attempts.

3. Tom plays by himself very well. His speech-language appear to be developing normally.

4. Sam and his parents look at books, play with picture cards, and listen to children's music and television shows together.

5. Sam's father plays "hop on pop" with Sam in which Sam climbs on his dad as Dad lies on the floor.

Mobilization Points:

1. Sam's mother is able to understand what Sam wants even if Sam doesn't use words to express himself.

2. Both parents enjoy playing with toys with Sam and use these times as opportunities to stimulate Sam's language.

3. Both parents use a technique in which they point to their mouths and say "tell me" when Sam doesn't use words to communicate. He sometimes responds by saying a word or two or by repeating "tell me" and then saying a word.

4. Sam imitates words over 50% of the time. His parents use this by asking a question, answering the question, and cheering for Sam when he imitates the word.

> Parent: What's this Sam?
> Parent: That's a car.
> Sam: That car.
> Parent: Good, Sam. That's a car, good for you! Yea!

5. When the parents don't know what Sam wants, they say "show me" and Sam sometimes points to the object.

6. Sam likes to sit by his mother as she looks at books and names the pictures for Sam.

7. The parents name things for Sam more than they ask him questions about the names of objects.

Speech-Language Characteristics:

1. Sam rarely spontaneously initiates verbal interaction in any form whether it be naming objects, pictures, or people; expressing a need; or greeting people. He says "no" in situations in which he is verbally stimulated, as if to mean "stop."

2. Sam communicates negation by saying "no."

3. We were unable to obtain reliable pointing responses to pictures or objects he named. The parents reported no better success.

4. It is difficult to achieve a shared focus of attention with Sam.

5. Sam attends to the details of toys (eg., the wheel of a toy tractor) and tends to "study" these rather than play with toys symbolically.

6. Sam did not interact visually with his parents during the session.

Initial Goal:

To develop nonverbal social interactions with Sam as a basis for communication.

First Assignment:

1. Notice the extent to which you are able to join Sam in a shared activity (eg., playing with toys) and the extent to which he will join you when you initiate the activity. Next week we'll talk about the times when this worked best.

  2. You do an excellent job of encouraging Sam to communicate. Keep doing these things.

  In this case, there was an obvious discrepancy between the parents' stated view of the problem and our view. Although the parents framed the problem in terms of their inability to understand Sam's speech, their efforts to help him were nearly all designed to encourage language usage. This discrepancy was discussed, and his parents agreed with our initial goal even though they were under the impression that the goal could be achieved quickly.

  Because of the difference in opinions, a "noticing assignment" was given for the first week rather than an intervention type of assignment. However, the parents were complimented for the excellent techniques that they had developed to help Sam use language, and they were encouraged to continue those activities. They were asked to bring one or two of Sam's books and some favorite toys to the next session to demonstrate their observations about establishing a shared focus of attention with Sam.

FAMILY NUMBER FOUR

Present at the first session: Maude, 77 years; husband, Earl
Chief Complaint: Maude's speech is slow; her memory is poor; and she has a moderate dysnomia following a stroke.
Family Characteristics and Interactions:

  1. Earl and Maude communicate in a friendly, cooperative, respectful manner.
  2. Much of what they talk about consists of functional matters, their adult children and grandchildren, and about events that occurred in their earlier life.
  3. The couple has two adult daughters and a son, all of whom live in different parts of the country, not near their parents.
  4. Earl appears to be in good health and drives; Maude has never driven.
  5. Earl and Maude have well-defined roles. Earl is retired and tends to the car, chores outside the house, and driving Maude to hair appointments, etc. He has always been helpful to Maude, but Maude was responsible for cooking, washing dishes, cleaning the house, and washing clothes.

Mobilization Points:
1. Earl usually knows the words that Maude has difficulty recalling; he often says them in an non-intrusive manner as they converse.
2. Sometimes Earl provides Maude with cues to help her think of words that she is attempting to recall. Maude appears to appreciate this, and she often is able to recall the word with this assistance.
3. Earl is patient with Maude and does not hurry her; his manner is gentle.
4. Maude's rate of speech is slow, and Earl appears to match this style by also speaking in a slow rate as the two interact. Earl does this very naturally and comfortably.
5. The couple's adult children and their children take turns visiting Earl and Maude so that a family comes for a long weekend about every month.
6. One of the adult children has invited Maude and Earl to come and live near them in a retirement center. Maude and Earl are considering this.
7. The couple has a number of good friends, all couples. Maude still enjoys getting together with them but is concerned that she cannot entertain as she did in the past.

Speech-Language Characteristics:
1. Maude's most obviously difficulty in speaking is dysnomia.
2. Maude's rate of speaking is slow, but precise.
3. Maude's immediate memory is poor; she is oriented to time and place.
4. A swallowing evaluation showed that no special eating or food modifications were necessary.
5. Maude enjoys the presence of her husband and her adult children and converses with them.

Initial Goals:
1. To improve Maude's ability to recall the names of things.
2. To maintain and improve, as desired by Maude and Earl, the conversational flow between them and between Maude and friends, her adult children, and her grandchildren.
3. To speak as naturally as possible with grandchildren on the telephone and to become more familiar with topics of conversation that interest them.

First Assignment:

1. Earl, you effectively assist Maude to communicate both by providing word cues and by supplying the word. Pay attention to how you use both of these and, particularly, the types of cues you give her that seem most useful in helping Maude recall words she is searching for.
2. When visiting with friends, pay attention to what you do to help Maude be a contributor to the conversation.

SUMMARY

Perhaps the most challenging component of Family-Based Treatment is linking the clinician's expertise with the resources and style of the family. It is at this point in the process that the clinician begins to truly empower families. Four examples are provided to illustrate the connection between family and speech-language characteristics and first assignments. The translation of data to appropriate goals is the result of creative strategizing. The degree of success of the process becomes evident at the subsequent meeting with the family.

CHAPTER 5

CREATING ASSIGNMENTS

Each Family-Based Treatment session culminates in the creation of one or more assignments, based upon the clinician's professional judgment and the family members' expertise. In the individual model, assignments are given to further the efforts of the clinician. These are often given without thought as to whether their purpose is understood by family members, whether they will fit the family's style of interaction, or whether or not they are based upon family resources. These are typically "sent home" with the client and usually involve some kind of intervention such as practicing a set of words or phrases with the client.

When families participate in treatment, assignments are given to help them promote change within the communicative interactions of the natural environment. Successful assignments rely heavily upon the clinician's ability to listen and learn. The clinician must connect her understanding of the problem with that of the family's and develop a treatment plan that capitalizes upon the resources of the family. This connection not only enlists but maintains family participation. The family is often able to improve upon assignments and tailor them even more specifically to their own unique situation. Toward that end, we use three types of assignments.

THREE TYPES OF ASSIGNMENTS

Noticing Assignments

A noticing assignment usually begins with a word or phrase such as "Notice" or "Pay attention to" some particular aspect of communication or interactions. Some examples are the following: "Notice the way Mark uses past tense verbs and write down some examples."; "Pay attention to the situations in which Jack is most fluent, and we'll discuss these next time we meet."; and, to an adult client with dysarthria who attended sessions with his spouse, "Notice what you do to control the loudness of your voice."

Noticing assignments can be used in a variety of situations for a variety of purposes. One situation in which they are useful is when the clinician and family members want to learn more about the speech-language characteristics of the client. When discussing plurals, for example, it is not uncommon for family members not to know whether or not their child uses these. After discussing their use and listening for them during a session, a noticing assignment may be given for family members to notice their use by the child at home. Both the family and the clinician will benefit from this information. A family, for example, can be more effective in carrying out interventions when they are familiar with the circumstances in which they will be asked to intervene. The clinician, on the other hand, may learn the extent to which use of plurals is an appropriate goal area.

Another purpose of noticing assignments is for everyone to learn more about the behaviors and interactions of parents, siblings, the client, spouses, or other family members. This type of assignment may lead to a greater appreciation of resources about which family members had been only generally aware or to the previously unnoticed effect of environmental variables. An example of an assignment like this is, "Notice Jacob's successes in controlling or handling situations well, and we'll ask you to describe what you've noticed next time we meet." This assignment was given to the family of a young child who was disfluent. Jacob's parents had just noticed that their son was maturing in a positive way and that fluency might be improved when he had a degree of control over situations. Other examples are: "Pay attention to the 'pause time' after John finishes speaking and before someone else speaks"; "Pay attention to the situations in which you feel most joined with Janice (e.g., when she looks at you, smiles, or acknowledges you)"; "Notice the situations in which Amanda stays focused on tasks the longest"; and "Pay attention to what you do when Kate indicates that she wants something."

A noticing type of assignment is often given to family members to build upon something that they have brought up during the session. John's parents, in the above example, had noticed that John's stuttering seemed to be related to their rate of speech as well as to that of his older brother's. After discussing this and having them play with John while they attempted to slow their rate, it became apparent that even when they slowed their rate, they were all quick to talk the instant that John paused. We discussed this briefly in the few remaining minutes of the session, and we all agreed that the assignment might help them appreciate speaking rate as it occurred in natural circumstances. As is often the case, the family not only noticed their conversational turn-taking behaviors, but attempted to do something about them. Thus, a noticing assignment *became* an intervention assignment as the family developed a better understanding of factors related to their child's fluency. Such assignments frequently have the effect of changing the behavior of family members since their attention becomes focused on communication.

The assignment to "notice" may also help family members gain a new appreciation for the positive aspects of their member's behavior or even an appreciation for positive things that they are already doing to help. Noticing exceptions to the problem (e.g., Notice the times that Kimberly is most vocal, when she phonates and babbles most) can direct parents' attention to behaviors desired in a quiet infant or toddler whose communicative development has been slow. The information also may be used so that similar conditions may be arranged. Another example, "Pay attention to the times that Juan is most fluent" may be given to parents who have attended to every feature of their child's disfluencies but know little about the conditions that facilitate fluency. When family members grow in appreciation of their family member's and their own resources, they usually become even more effective partners in treatment.

One last example of noticing assignments is to call a client's attention to strategies he is using to help himself. We asked an adult with dysarthria who was struggling to speak in a quieter voice, to pay attention to what he was doing when he was successful in using a quiet voice. We asked his spouse to attend to any conditions that seemed to help her husband with this task. We also asked this client to pay attention to the techniques he used that helped him the most in situations where he particularly needed to be intelligible. He discovered, for himself, some things he was doing of which he had not been completely aware. The clinician used the information to suggest related techniques, and it added new information to his repertoire of strategies not only for this client but for future clients in similar circumstances.

The clinician's *intent* in developing and delivering an assignment is critical to the assignment's success. Giving a noticing assignment so that a family will discover how "bad" they are will not be successful! Rather, it will serve to alienate the family from the clinician and undermine the partnership. The clinician's intent must be to be helpful and to nudge the therapeutic process forward rather than to expose weaknesses of the family or to demonstrate the clinician's superiority.

Intervention Assignments

A second type of assignment is more traditional and involves assigning family members something overt to do or something to refrain from doing. We call this type of assignment an "intervention assignment" since it involves an overt action. Intervention assignments are made to alter the communicative environment of the client (1) by family members initiating interaction or responding to the client in a particular way or (2) by family members interacting among themselves in a particular manner. Some examples are as follows: "Use family photos to elicit past tense verbs and restate what Mark says using the correct form of the verb."; "Exaggerate the consonants in your own speech as you interact with Darin. This will call them to his attention much like a highlighter is used to call our visual attention to a printed word"; "I think you're right that asking David to say words isn't working. This week, when you look at books, you name things and point to them. Go slowly and pause so as to leave 'spaces' for him to talk if he wants to (eg., 'I see a ....car')."; "Listeners can understand you best when you exaggerate your articulation and the rhythm of your speech. Practice that this week in situations when you want to be particularly intelligible."

We think of intervention assignments as having three important ingredients. They should be *systemic, polyocular, and isomorphic.* Assignments are systemic when they may be carried out in the context of typical interactions by one or more family members. This is as opposed to assigning practice time, work time, or drilling time. Speech-language pathologists using an individual model of service delivery may work in this manner, but we do not suggest it as a method for families. Rather, the clinician should attempt to maintain the advantage of the natural environment by suggesting communication techniques that may be inserted into typical family interactions and modified to help the client. One way to insert practice into everyday interactions with children is to use a "stop and say" technique. This technique involves (1) "stopping" a child when he is not busily engaged in any other activity, (2) asking the child to "say" one selected word or phrase, (3) reinforcing a successful attempt, and (4) resuming the activity in which everyone was engaged prior to the intervention. We suggest that the activity be centered on words or sounds the child can be expected to say successfully, even if help is needed (e.g., the parent may exaggerate some aspect of the word or phrase), but if the child is not successful, the parent is advised to say nothing or something like "good try" and resume normal activities, not to ask the child to try again. This activity can occur as everyday activities are occurring: when the child enters the bathroom and the father is shaving, during a commercial on a television program, before or after reading a book to the child, when the child is in the tub, etc. It should not be attempted when the child is engaged in an activity or might otherwise be distracted from something in which she is interested.

A second characteristic of intervention assignments is that they are most successful when they are polyocular, that is, when the assignment is based upon the polyocular perspective described in Chapter 1. Everyone's view, including the clinician's, must be accommodated in the assignment for it to be successful. Further, assignments are understood best when they flow naturally from the discussion and activities in which the family was engaged during the session. After the previous assignment has been reviewed, for example, the clinician is likely to have one or more ideas for a subsequent suggestion that builds upon the first. The clinician may try out the new idea or explain it to the family and ask them to try it out along with the clinician's "coaching." A discussion of the strategy usually follows. Topics discussed include: the response of the client, the degree of difficulty in using the strategy for the family members, and the extent to which the activity could fit into the family's daily activities. In this way, the assignment is not a surprise but rather a natural activity that has been discussed, practiced, and perhaps modified.

Third, intervention assignments are most successful when they are *isomorphic* to the family; for example, they consist of activities similar to those in which family members typically engage. We would not, for example, give an assignment to read a book to a father who usually interacts with his child by playing with toys and creating imaginative play situations. Nor would we ask a spouse to give her husband cues to assist him in recalling the names of objects when he is helping her cook if they have never cooked together in the entire forty-five years of their marriage. Rather, we would suggest that interventions be carried out, in the first example, as the father and child play; in the second, we would choose a typical interactive activity in which the couple engages.

Assessing Effectiveness of Assignments

A third type of assignment is given to assess the results of particular interventions and of the overall treatment plan. These are called "assessing effectiveness" assignments. Some examples are as follows: "Listen to find out whether or not Mark spontaneously revises sentences to use the correct verb form."; "Julie is beginning to hold brief 'conversations' with you. Write down some examples of these in a script form."; and "Write down words that you hear Gretchen say spontaneously this week."

The clinician may compare the information derived from "assessing effectiveness" assignments to the behavior observed during the session.

Family members can point out similarities to what they have heard at home or in some cases describe the differences between the client's home behavior and that elicited during the session. This provides additional data to be combined with other information gained during the session in order to develop the next assignment. The information may also be used to highlight the role and ability of family members to stimulate change in the client.

Assignments are the clinician's link to change. The success or failure of treatment hinges on the appropriateness of assignments and the manner in which assignments are delivered.

SUCCESS AND FAILURE OF ASSIGNMENTS

Assignments of any type must consist of activities in which everyone involved can be successful. First, the client must be able to do whatever is being asked of her. We never give an assignment for families to ask the client to do something that we have not seen her do with some ease during the session. We remind parents to keep their child successful at least 80% of the time. That is, eight out of ten times they ask their child to do something, she must do it successfully. Family members are shown how to revert to a simpler level of activity if they find that the child's success level is falling below 80%. The same is true when we work with adults and have spouses, adult children, etc. use techniques to facilitate communication during conversation.

Not only must the client be successful, but also the family members doing the intervention. We keep the 80% rule in mind for families, too, although we seldom phrase it that way to them. When we discover that an assignment is too difficult for family members to do, we change it before they leave the session. We want very much to send families home with tasks that both they and the client can complete successfully.

Following is a brief illustration of this principle. Eric was 54 months old and had been born with a bilateral cleft lip and palate. We had seen Eric and his family when he was 30 months old and worked to establish a variety of places of articulation. At 40 months, our goals had been met, but Eric was still quite hypernasal. We agreed to take a break from treatment until anticipated pharyngeal flap surgery was completed. This proved to be more than a year away. Eric's father called after obtaining clearance from the plastic surgeon that speech-language treatment could proceed without doing damage to the new surgically placed pharyngeal flap. At the first session, Eric somehow managed to have nasal air emission on every production of /s/ and on most productions of other voiceless sibilants. Eric's father and Jim worked with Eric for forty minutes without obtaining an oral air stream for any sibilant. Eric could, however, produce a strongly aspirated /t/ in isolation (or, at least when paired with a whispered neutral vowel). This became the assignment even though Jim very much wanted to send Eric and his father home to practice /s/ as produced with an oral air stream. This was not, however, possible for Eric to do and would only lead to frustration for him, his father and mother, and likely his siblings. Eric and his father left with the assignment to elicit strongly aspirated /t/ sounds; his father was to verbally praise Eric when he did this. They planned to do it for very short periods of time (one to two minutes) when *both* were "in the mood," and Eric's father assured Jim that he could keep the practice enjoyable for both of them.

As to the outcome at the next session, Eric came back producing /s/ with an oral air stream. This was fortuitous and occurred as Eric's father created a variety of enjoyable games that made it possible for his son to change. It is not, however, the point of the illustration. The point is this: assignments must consist of activities with which both family members and clients can be successful. The alternative is to have discouraged, frustrated families returning grudgingly for the next session (until they give up and start missing appointments).

DELIVERING THE ASSIGNMENT

The single most important factor in delivering an assignment is the clinician's intent. The clinician who has a genuinely helpful intention for each assignment is unable to hide this from families. Similarly, families recognize the intentions of clinicians who give assignments designed to uncover the family's ineptness, incomplete knowledge, and/or inadequacy. The clinician with good intentions may give an inappropriate assignment but at worst, the family reports that they were unable to complete it. The clinician who highlights a family's negative features, is unlikely to learn the results of assignments since family members will probably react by withdrawing and devaluing their resources.

Second, it is most appropriate to deliver the assignment by making reference to something that the family has already mentioned, something that has been previously discussed with the family, or something that occurred during the session that was pertinent. In other words, successful assignments are *isomorphic* to the family's view of reality and will fit into their daily routine of activities. It is also helpful for families to view the assignment in context, that is as an integral part of the total treatment plan rather than as an isolated act. Appropriate assignments should follow in such a tight, logical order that families are not surprised by the next step. However, it is helpful for the clinician to make this sequential connection when delivering the assignment.

Third, assignments are most likely to be successful when they are linked with positive actions already being accomplished by family members. As an assignment is being planned, it is good time to evaluate the family's contribution to the progress that the client is making. Because the clinician attempts to identify those things that family members do well, it is natural to reinforce the particular efforts of families in conjunction with delivering the next assignment. For example, "Allen is responding well to your efforts to say words to him rather than asking him to talk. I know it's difficult, but you're doing it well. This week, try pausing some of the time when you are looking at the book with him; say a partial sentence and pause. If he doesn't say the word, you go ahead and say it and go on looking at the book. You're doing an excellent job of not asking him questions."

Fourth, the clinician should ask the family whether or not they think the assignment is possible to do and if they think it will be effective. Usually they will respond positively; sometimes, however, they have concerns about it. When this occurs, use listening skills to determine what is concerning them and modify the assignment or give a new one. It is very important that family members understand the assignment and believe that they will be able to carry it out.

Fifth, the clinician should demonstrate the assignment and then ask members of the family to try it during the session. This allows the family to see exactly what is being asked of them and lets everyone in the session see his or her member's response. This is followed by family members practicing the assignment. The clinician can then observe the client's responses to the family as compared with those elicited that he elicited. As might be expected, the client usually responds better to members of her family than to the clinician. This allows the clinician to emphasize the familial bond, and again, reinforcing the family. As family members carry out the assignment, the clinician can also critically evaluate their performance and give them feedback. Reward those things that they do well and suggest modifications of behaviors that could be improved. This should be done as family members are carrying out the assignment so that they have the opportunity to try again immediately and to ask for additional assistance if the client seems not to be responsive.

Finally, after talking about the assignment, the clinician should provide it for the family in writing. Our format for assignments includes the date, the names of those present, reinforcing remarks, the specific assignment(s), and the date/time of the next session. A copy of the form is included in Appendix B.

FAMILY RESPONSES TO ASSIGNMENTS

In most cases, the assignment is delivered; families show they are capable of performing the tasks assigned; and the next appointment is scheduled. In others, however, family members may respond unenthusiastically to the assignment or indicate their dislike for it. Families with whom the clinical partnership is strong tell the clinician almost immediately when they disagree with assignments and when assignments do not fit their family style. The manner of response varies with families. With some family members it is direct and with others it may be limited to a skeptical look and a few questions. The clinician should attend carefully to nonverbal responses in order to discuss modifications with the client and family. We want their feedback to assure us that we have developed suggestions that they will be comfortable doing.

We always elicit feedback about assignments during the session at which they are given. We attempt to do it in such a way that we invite even the most reluctant family member to express a genuine opinion. "What do you think of this? Is this something that you think you can do comfortably? Do you think it will make a difference?"

On rare occasions, family members may appear to be hostile, defensive, or indifferent as they respond to assignments. These responses tell us that we must do something different. Eddie and his family illustrate this principle nicely. Eddie was an active four-year-old only child who came with his mother and father. The father was the spokesperson for the family and cared for Eddie during the day. Eddie's speech was approximately 60% intelligible, and his parents were concerned. Further, it was difficult to obtain Eddie's cooperation to administer an articulation test and to determine exactly the nature of his speech problem.

For several weeks, Eddie's father and mother exaggerated the designated consonants in their own speech as they interacted with Eddie and reinforced him when he said words clearly. This intervention was proceeding successfully, but the observation team who watched the sessions from behind a one-way mirror had some other suggestions for Jim and a student to take back to the treatment room. The two clinicians were pleased with the team's suggestions and described them to the parents. To the clinician's surprise, Eddie's father responded negatively. "Has Eddie not been improving?" he asked. "Why change things when he's making progress?" Eddie's father's position was that Eddie was making positive changes; therefore, we should not move too fast in our work, but rather keep making steady, reliable progress and not change anything. And, we didn't; we kept everything the same. At subsequent sessions, Jim and the student used phrases such as, "We'll take this one step at a time;" "We'll build on what we know works and keep things moving;" and "Let's keep doing what works and not risk unsuccessful side trips." Eddie did keep improving, the slow, steady way! Not by our choice, but most importantly, by his parent's choice.

SUMMARY

The activities of each session are directed toward the development and delivery of an assignment that will promote speech-language improvement in the family member with a communicative disorder. Successful assignments are systemic in nature in that they are to be carried out during natural interactions. While attempts are made to match the assignment with the style of the family and take into account factors such as roles, rules, and hierarchy, families are expected to modify the assignment to make for a better "fit" as they carry out the activities. This is natural and possible when family members understand the purpose of the assignment and the goal toward which it is directed.

Three types of assignments are available to the clinician. One is a *noticing assignment*, given for family members to learn more about the problem, for the clinician to learn more about the family and/or the client, or to strengthen a new insight or perception that family members express. A second type of assignment is an *intervention assignment*, one in which family members are directed to do something or not to do something. Finally, an *assessing effectiveness assignment* is given to determine the effect of the treatment program or to call family members' attention to change that has occurred.

Assignments are most successful when they are delivered in the spirit of good intentions, when everyone can be successful in their implementation, and when the clinician relates them to existing information with which the family is familiar. Further, assignments are most effective when they are explained in the context of reinforcement, when family members are invited to comment upon their appropriateness, and when they are demonstrated by the clinician and practiced by the family.

CHAPTER 6

ASSESSING TREATMENT EFFECTIVENESS

Significantly more time is given to the process step of "assessing treatment effectiveness" than to any other step in the Family-Based Treatment process. The skill with which the clinician has completed the earlier steps, however, pre-determines the success of this one. Families have more than a first impression by the time the clinician is assessing the effectiveness of the assignments that have been delivered. Important accomplishments include, but are not limited to factors such as: the degree to which a family-clinician partnership is underway; the quality of information the clinician and family have shared; and the extent to which the clinician has combined everyone's expertise, including his own; and the success of the early assignment(s), for client and family members alike.

ASSESSING TREATMENT

We begin with the assumption that, initially, we will meet with a family once per week for one hour. Typically, when positive change is starting to occur after several sessions, the time between sessions is lengthened by mutual agreement to every other week. Later, we may agree to meet every three weeks or even once per month.

The typical pattern of a session is as follows: (1) briefly review the goals of treatment; (2) discuss in detail, using counseling techniques (see Chapter 8), the assignment from the previous session; (3) have family members demonstrate or enact the assignment if it involves using a behavioral technique; (4) when appropriate, enact the assignment ourselves and experiment with modifying it or using new interventions, in order to determine how to promote further change; (5) have family members carry out the new technique or style of interaction; and, (6) discuss the new assignment. Not every session follows this identical plan, but it is the format from which we depart. In this manner, the effectiveness of treatment is assessed, and modifications are made in the interest of promoting change as quickly as possible.

Review the Goals of Treatment

Family members have already participated in setting treatment goals and have agreed upon them. Their understanding of these, however, may be less complete than that of the clinician since most family members are not accustomed to thinking in detail about communicative behavior. Further, the link between the assignment and the goals may be unclear. When the latter seems the case, it is helpful to talk about the goal(s) and the procedures together. For example, in a second session we restated the goal as follows: "Our goal is to improve Robert's intelligibility. We all noticed that when he uses more effort, talks louder, and emphasizes the stress and rhythm of his speech, he is much easier to understand. In an effort to encourage him to do this, you have been emphasizing the rhythm of your own speech as you interact with him. You also do this as you repeat some of the words and phrases that he says to you. Your doing these things calls them to his attention and makes it more likely that he, too, will speak in this manner. Another thing you do is to reinforce Robert when he uses more effort and emphasizes the rhythm of his speech. You let him know that you're pleased, and you comment that you can understand him really well."

The example of Robert was taken from the second session with him and his family. Robert had a genetic defect that resulted in mental retardation. He was nine years old. His family included the following members: his father; his stepmother; and his stepbrother, the thirteen-year-old son of his stepmother. Robert lived with his father's family most of the time. His family also included his natural mother and his mother's friend. Robert visited his mother's family on weekends. Everyone attended the treatment sessions. All these people were interested in Robert and were willing to help him. Their cooperation and participation was positively framed in terms of how fortunate Robert was to have all of his family participating and to have many people who cared about him.

Review the Assignment

It is important to use neutral questioning to learn how family members carry out assignments. At Robert's third session, for example, we asked, "What happened when you exaggerated the rhythm of your speech as you interacted with Robert?" Our assumption was that the assignment had been carried out. Had it not been, family members could have said that they did not do it, that it was unsuccessful, that they modified it, etc. more readily than if our question had been the more accusatory, "Did you do the assignment?" Since it is critical to know the family's response to assignments, any techniques that lead to elaboration and discussion are useful. The role of the clinician is to match his expertise with each family's resources and capabilities in order to effect change in the family member having the communicative problem. When the assignment is not carried out in any fashion whatsoever, it is important to know the reason so that a more appropriate assignment can be given. When families change or modify the assignment, we do not view this as a failure. In many cases, the modification improves upon the assignment and makes it "fit" more closely to interaction patterns of the family. In other cases, the assignment may have been misinterpreted or not clearly understood. It is, therefore, important that the clinician listen, track, and clarify in order to learn exactly what happened when the assignment was attempted. Once the family's efforts have been explored, they can show the clinician what they did. This gives an even better understanding of the effectiveness of the assignment and allows the clinician to modify it or expand upon it appropriately.

To continue with the example of Robert, his stepmother answered first when we asked what happened when they carried out the assignment. She described many examples of exaggerating the rhythm of her speech. She did this when making cookies with Robert, imitating a person they saw on television, talking with Robert as he arrived home from school each day, putting Robert to bed, eating meals, and interacting in the course of daily living. Tracking was used to learn exactly what happened; this allowed the clinician to develop visual images of the technique being used. The clinician asked about where in the house the technique was used, what each person said in the dialog, how each reacted emotionally to the assignment in terms of ease and enjoyment, and the extent to which Robert changed his speech during the interaction. Other examples were given by Robert's father and his step-brother. Robert's natural mother modified the assignment slightly in order to make it fit her activities with her son. She carried out the assignment when singing songs with Robert and when reading books to him. She described exactly what had happened, and we asked her to look at a book with Robert during the session and show us what she did. While requests for enactments could be interpreted as skepticism on the clinician's part, when this is done out of genuine curiosity and interest, we have not found families to be defensive. More often, they enjoy showing us what they have done. Those interactions that look especially favorable are discussed and reinforced. When young children are involved, we particularly like to respond to the parent by reacting positively to the parent-child relationship in terms of the child's response to the parent and/or the parent's particular manner of interacting with the child. We also reinforce family behavior that shows enjoyment of communicating and interacting with the client. This is done by amplifying the positive things we notice.

Sometimes family members' initial responses to the clinician's inquiry about what happened when they did the assignment is cursory and incomplete. When parents of a four- year-old who omitted /k/ sounds was asked what happened when they exaggerated the /k/ sound in their own speech, the father answered, "Not much." Had the clinician accepted this answer and not probed further, a good deal of information would have been lost. Rather, tracking (Chapter 8) was used to learn exactly when each parent exaggerated the sound, where they were when they did it, and what they were doing when they did it. During this process, the child leaned into a microphone that allowed observers to hear as they watched in an adjacent room and exaggerated each /k/ as she said, "Cookie." Both parents expressed surprise and agreed that she had not done this at home. After we all praised the child and enjoyed the irony of the moment together, the parents added that they had not only exaggerated the sound as they said it in words, but that they had also said the sound in isolation many times when they were in the presence of the child. They continued with a story about an event in which the child "said /k/, /k/, /k/, /k/ with each step as she walked around the living room." This was followed by a description by the father of making up stories with the child and finding excuses to include many words that had included the /k/ sound. All this followed the cursory answer of "Not much" and would have been lost had the issue not been probed in detail. Tracking exactly what family members did as they carried out assignments, sometimes yields information that changes the course of treatment even when, initially, nothing significant is reported.

Enact the Assignment and Develop a New One

Since most communicative change occurs outside of treatment sessions when the Family-Based Treatment model is used, it is necessary for clinicians to determine the extent to which change has occurred so that appropriate new assignments may be developed. One technique for doing this is to ask family members to *show* the clinician what they did and the gains that the client has made. This is usually done in a natural relaxed manner when family members have participated in the initial assessment and are accustomed to demonstrating their activities for the clinician. In addition, of course, the family has observed as the clinician demonstrated additional techniques and evaluated these in terms of the ease with which they could be accomplished at home. Problem-solving *together* is an important part of the clinician-family partnership. The clinician typically enters the situation not knowing exactly what the new assignment will be, but with confidence that a new assignment will emerge as he engages in discussion and experimentation, while adopting a polyocular perspective. One thing I (Jim) discovered when I began working with families was that I didn't have to work as hard as when I used an individual treatment approach. My knowledge and expertise seemed to be maximized when I allowed (invited) families to help me determine the course of action to take. The responsibility is not mine alone, but rather, the responsibility is shared with family members. Together, I know, that we will develop an assignment that will work better for the family and the client than the one I alone would have developed.

Continuing with the description of Robert's family, after they described their activities and enacted the assignment, we interacted with Robert and began experimenting by calling Robert's attention to specific sounds and sound groups while emphasizing the rhythm of speech. Since Robert did not always close his lips for bilabial sounds and because exaggerating the rhythm of speech seemed to facilitate lip closure, several minutes were spent in an effort to determine the feasibility of an assignment that would incorporate attending particularly to bilabial sounds in the context of increased loudness and rhythm. We practiced words such as "mama, mine, boy, pie." Robert's family began adding words that they knew would come up during the week, and we discussed the possibility of adding a list of specific words containing /b/, /p/, and /m/ to the assignment of overall exaggerated use of loudness variation and rhythm. Robert's family began asking Robert to imitate family-related words (i.e., words associated with family experiences). This gave us the opportunity to observe how such an assignment would be carried out at home. His family members reinforced Robert's attempts appropriately, and we commented about the importance of doing this and their ability to do so. We discussed whether or not attending to all three phonemes would be too difficult for Robert and for the family and decided that it would not be. A list of ten words and phrases based upon words said at home was developed for practice. Correct imitation was defined as lip approximation; this was to be rewarded. The previous week's assignment was also continued since it had been successful in improving Robert's intelligibility.

It was suggested that the ten specific words be practiced during normal everyday activities. A "stop and say" activity, which we have used successfully with a number of families, was described. In this activity, the practice word is said to the client by a family member in the course of natural interactions such as when eating dinner, when entering the same room, while watching television, etc. The family member says the word, the family member with the speech-language problem repeats it, success is reinforced, and natural activities are resumed. Most families make an enjoyable activity out of this and find it to be an easy way to incorporate structured speech practice into everyday events. In addition, since the word list contained words and phrases that were known to be part of family conversation, it was expected that use of the words would arise out of natural interactions.

This same "stop and say" activity may be used to practice plurals, verb tense, possessiveness, slow easy speech, and nearly any other aspect of verbal communication. One parent, practicing plurals with her child, stopped the child and said "One duck, . . . two . . .?" whereupon she paused and the child said, "Two ducks." The noun was changed to other words, some rather silly, which kept the child's interest and increased the enjoyment of the activity. Soon, plurals were used in conversation. The child's attention was heightened by using some of the same words that had been used during the "stop and say" technique and maintaining the spirit of fun as conversations evolved. This facilitated the child's use of plurals rather quickly.

Have Family Members Practice the New Assignment

It is very useful to observe family members as they carry out new assignments. Their understanding of the suggestion may be very different than the clinician's, even when both have used the same words to describe it. The mutual understanding that seems very clear may not actually exist. For example, even though it may appear to be easy to follow a child's lead during play and to make comments rather than ask questions, it may be surprisingly difficult for family members to do this. Exaggerating the rhythm of speech or stressing consonant sounds may look easy when the clinician demonstrates for the family. It may prove to be so unnatural to some family members that it is not the good suggestion it initially seemed to be.

In the case of one family with whom we worked, the family agreed, after watching the clinician, that following the child's lead during play and describing what the child was doing, rather than asking questions, was an effective technique. The time for ending the session was approaching, and since everyone seemed to be in agreement and understood what to do, we considered omitting the step of asking family members to practice. When we decided to take a few minutes for family members to quickly practice, we realized that the assignment, as planned, was not likely to be successful. It was very difficult for family members to refrain from asking questions. As the father played with the child, he made very few comments and asked many questions. When we noticed this, we smiled as we looked at the other family members who notified the father that he was asking questions rather than making comments. He suggested, "This is harder than it looks!" They all agreed. Their solution was to "correct" one another; they all agreed that this would be an enjoyable way to implement this assignment that looked easy but which, in reality, introduced a different way of playing and interacting with their child than they were accustomed to using. They spent a short time practicing the assignment, as modified. They described it as "catching" each other asking questions. We were assured that this could be done in the spirit of fun and agreed that if they disliked this manner of completing the assignment, they would discontinue doing it until our next session. In less than five minutes, we modified an assignment, with the help of the family, that would not have resulted in the communicative change we all wanted even when it appeared that everyone understood exactly how the assignment should be carried out. This, of course, was a healthy, playful family. They suggested a modification that would not be successful in some other families. In this case, the clinician did not determine how to solve the problem, the family did. Their suggestion was idiosyncratic to their interactive style and made the original assignment one that would be a challenging, but enjoyable family activity. The step of discussing the assignment was short, but effective.

Discuss the New Assignment with the Family

A good deal of discussion of the new assignment typically has taken place already as the assignment is developed and practiced. Once the assignment is at that stage, we put it in writing and give it to the family (Appendix C). They usually read it quickly, we confirm one last time that they are in agreement with the plan, and ask if they have any questions. This last bit of business at the end of the session allows the family to think seriously about what they will be doing, and it allows the clinician an opportunity to add or emphasize aspects of the assignment as seems appropriate. In the case of the above example, the clinician might confirm once more that if listening to "catch" another family member asking questions starts to be more offensive than fun, that they stop and wait until we have more time to practice during the next session. In the case of a parent who asked his child to say many words that the child was unable to say precisely, we had suggested that eight out of ten times the child should be able to respond requests successfully. Even though we spent an entire session outlining the circumstances in which the child could be successful and practiced intermixing "easy" words with "difficult" words, we reviewed the "eighty percent rule" one last time before the family left the session. Potential assignments should be discussed as they are being developed and practiced. This final step provides one more opportunity for all participants to confirm their confidence in and understanding of the new assignment.

EXPECTING POSITIVE CHANGE

Sometimes in the context of treatment, clinicians, including us, temporarily lose sight of the original desire for communicative change that was present in earlier sessions with a family. Sessions become routine, assignments lack insight and may not be tailored for an isomorphic family fit, family perspectives are forgotten or are placed in the background, and our zest for change becomes lackluster. This is a temporary setback rather than a typical style of operation, and it can occur to clinicians and families alike as treatment progresses.

We know of no ideal solution to this situation other than reminding ourselves prior to sessions that we very much want change to occur. I (Jim) remind myself that I want this client to change as much as Michael Jordan wanted the Chicago Bulls to win the basketball game. This internal pep talk might be insufficient for some; for others, however, it may serve as a reminder that our work is of greater importance to each particular client and family member than a basketball victory. I (Mary) remember to ". . . approach each session as if it were the last and only time you will see that client" (Walter & Peller, 1992, pp. 40). This helps me stay intensely focused on creating change in each session. Our original goal of Family-Based Treatment was to create change quickly. With some families, this has occurred and in ten sessions or fewer a speech-language difficulty has been resolved. In others, the communicative disorder is part of a general condition that will be long-term, or even life-long. Even in the latter cases, we have found the systemic, family-centered, solution-focused principles to be effective because families become empowered to use new interventions, to celebrate their involvement in creating small change, and to balance hope with reality.

SUMMARY

The activities described above provide an example of the manner in which treatment effectiveness can be assessed in each session. Treatment sessions consist of six broad steps from which departures occur as appropriate to promote the therapeutic process. The primary goal of this step in the Family-Based Treatment process is to assess the effects of treatment and to make additional suggestions that will nudge the process of change forward as quickly as possible. When an assignment has not been carried out, neutral questioning should be used to determine what happened. Depending on the results of that discussion, the assignment may be re-delivered, adjusted, or discarded. When assessing the results of an assignment, the clinician should use tracking as well as listening and other counseling techniques to determine exactly what happened, when it happened and where. In our experience, when family members participate in assessing the results of what they are doing, there is less likelihood that ineffective procedures will be continued beyond a week or two. Family members usually know whether or not their activities are promoting change and are eager to alter them when they are not. When families are allowed to be full participants on the treatment team, both the clinician and family members are freed to communicate honestly and respectfully about the value of treatment procedures.

CHAPTER 7

TERMINATING AND LINKING

A decision to end treatment must be made at some point in the Family-Based Treatment process. We have used four different options to end therapy with our families: a last session scheduled at the end of a predetermined number of sessions, gradual spacing of sessions leading to a mutual decision to terminate as family members assume responsibility for intervention, termination following a one or two session consultation, and linking to other professionals who continue treatment with the client. A combination of methods may be used based upon the combined wisdom of the family and the clinician.

Defined Number of Sessions

A variety of circumstances may lead the clinician and family to designate a defined number of sessions at the outset. The length of treatment, such as six total sessions over a period of six weeks, is known by all participants when treatment begins. Some examples are the following: summer sessions with children who will be returning to school services in the fall, family sessions at short and long-term medical facilities that end when the patient is transferred to another facility or goes home, or a limited number of family sessions organized to fit the busy schedules of both the clinician and the family. This kind of termination may be as dependent on the clinician's professional options as it is on the family's availability. At the final session, accomplishments are highlighted, and the family members are complimented for their participation. If the client will be continuing services with another speech-language pathologist, we include that person in the final session to assure a smooth transition.

Gradual Spacing of Sessions

When families are empowered participants in treatment, it is not unusual to reduce the frequency of meetings after several sessions and after the clinician is confident that family members are intervening effectively. This is especially true when the communicative disorder is one that is expected to change slowly through a combination of treatment and maturation. Complete termination of treatment is usually inappropriate in such cases and may be replaced with bi-weekly or monthly sessions with the family. Even longer intervals may be planned. An important aspect of such a decision is that it be made mutually with the family. We often call the longer break a "vacation" and schedule a follow-up meeting four to six months after the last regular meeting so that progress can be monitored.

It is significant to note that treatment interventions are continuing during this time even though the speech-language pathologist is not meeting with the family. The family has learned to build speech-language change into its everyday life and is maintaining the gains achieved during family treatment. The signal that longer intervals between meetings might be appropriate is that the clinician finds that the creative strategizing process does not lead to a significant alteration in the assignments. Naturally, the clinician assumes that family members are continuing to intervene during these breaks. We find this to be a valid assumption when family members are an integral part of the solution-focused treatment team. At the follow-up meeting, progress is monitored, developmental change assessed, and the possibility of scheduling another series of sessions is discussed.

One or Two Session Consultation

Many clinicians have heavy caseloads and are not able to work with families on an ongoing basis. One or two consultation sessions may be arranged with families so that the clinician's schedule does not become overcrowded. A school conference is an example of this kind of meeting. Even though the time is short, the Family-Based Treatment process and techniques may be used to develop partnerships with families.

In addition, clinicians who work systemically are likely to be called upon by families for one or two-session consultations. Families who request this are not seeking assessment and treatment in the usual sense; rather, they want the speech-language pathologist's opinion about a communicative problem and/or suggestions for ways to improve interaction with a family member having a communicative disorder. Termination of services is expected after the number of agreed-upon sessions has been completed.

Linking With Other Professionals

The process of linking with other professionals is an intervention that can be used to facilitate the family's continuing involvement in services. It is not unusual for several professionals and even several speech-language pathologists to become involved when treatment begins with a very young child. Over time, the treatment team may expand to include many different teachers, school and clinical psychologists, parent interventionists, occupational therapists, physical therapists, school administrators, rehabilitation counselors, social workers, and speech-language pathologists. Treatment becomes significantly more complicated as the need to share and integrate data expands with the addition of each new professional. The speech-language pathologist's treatment in many of these cases should include linking the families with other professionals in a way that advances and maintains the families as integral decision-makers on the treatment team. The clinician can facilitate this process in several ways. These include showing that she respects the family's views in transition meetings, talking about the communicative problem as it manifests itself interactively, describing the interventions that family members have carried out, and having family members demonstrate their skills to team members.

The clinician must respect the views of the other professionals on the team just as she respects the views of the family. She should identify professional resources and search for points of agreement, just as she does when working with the family alone. Her intent is to link the family to other professional resources in a positive way.

SUMMARY

Four different options have been described relative to ending Family-Based Treatment. Two of these are variations of agreed-upon or implied short-term treatment or consultation. Not all families with a member with a communicative disorder need or desire more than a few sessions with a speech-language pathologist or audiologist. In some cases a family may want the opinion of the speech-language pathologist about the severity of a problem, the need for treatment, or about suggestions for activities that could be carried out at home. With other families, services are more traditionally oriented, and termination is not pre-determined. When treatment is long-term and the client is young, maturation may be a factor in change, and breaks in treatment may be arranged. If termination leads to services that are provided by another professional person, it is important to link the family with the appropriate person or persons and clarify the anticipated level of family participation in a positive way.

CHAPTER 8

COUNSELING TECHNIQUES

Family participation in the treatment of communicative disorders is most effective when counseling techniques are integrated into the entire treatment process. We do not think of counseling as an adjunct to therapy set aside as a separate process from the evaluation and treatment of speech-language-hearing problems. Rather, we suggest that counseling be defined as the use of a set of techniques that enables the clinician to respond to client and family statements, behaviors, and interactions in a manner that expands clinical effectiveness and enhances speech-language change. In this chapter we will discuss the integrated use of counseling techniques, describe the techniques that are used in Family-Based Treatment, and outline the issues and counseling responses associated with the grieving process.

AN INTEGRATED APPROACH TO COUNSELING

When counseling techniques are integrated into speech-language treatment, they permeate the entire treatment process. Consider a metaphor that illustrates this perspective. When preparing a subtly flavored tomato sauce, to be served with fresh pasta, the basil that is added to the sauce does not settle in one area and affect only that part of the sauce; instead, it permeates the entire culinary creation and changes the flavor of the sauce as well as the completed pasta-sauce entree. Like the herbs in a tomato sauce, counseling techniques added to the treatment process permeate and enhance the clinician's work. The clinician's continuing use of these techniques "flavors" the process in a way that changes the totality of the clinician-family relationship and profoundly effects the outcome of treatment. Further, these techniques are not reserved for "problem situations" but are used to enhance every aspect of speech-language treatment.

We integrate counseling techniques into all aspects of Family-Based Treatment and cannot predict, specifically, when they will be used; however, there are several situations that may lead the clinician to use the techniques. These include activities such as enlisting family cooperation and participation; interviewing clients and family members to obtain diagnostic and other information; presenting assessment results, especially unwelcome information; responding to emotions that are expressed by clients and/or family members; communicating with co-workers, supervisors, and supervisees; and problem solving with professionals from different treatment orientations. A discussion of each of these situations follows.

Enlisting Family Participation

We are continually working to develop a partnership relationship with our clients and their families. Most family members approach the family-centered experience eager to participate in this process. Some family members, however, may show disinterest, hostility, or other behaviors that seem to signal an unwillingness to participate. These behaviors usually change as the clinician adopts a polyocular perspective and shows respect for the divergent views expressed. Many of the families referred to us have been identified as "uncooperative" by one or more professionals. The use of counseling techniques, along with the assumption that each family member cares deeply for his family member with a communicative disorder, helps us move quickly to a partnership relationship.

Our thinking about cooperative partnerships has been influenced by the work of Steve deShazer, a family therapist from Milwaukee, Wisconsin (1985). He and his team of family therapists discovered the family's style of cooperating by analyzing the responses of their clients to assigned tasks and then creating subsequent tasks that more closely approximated the family's response. deShazer assumed that if family members do not cooperate with the therapist, the therapist has failed to develop a task that fits the family's style of cooperating. The team must then request behavior that fits the family's natural patterns of interaction more closely. Speech-language pathologists who shift to a systemic way of thinking (see Chapter 1) and who use the techniques described in this chapter should be able to enlist family members as cooperative partners on the treatment team.

Interviewing Clients and Family Members to Obtain Diagnostic and Other Information

As the reader no doubt knows, a well-conducted interview produces useful diagnostic information. When counseling techniques are integrated into the interview, diagnostic information is obtained that is often more in-depth than that obtained from a traditional interview. Also, new ideas related to treatment options begin to emerge as the clinician encourages the client and family members to share their knowledge and resources.

Presenting Assessment Results, Especially Unwelcome Information

Speech-language pathologists and audiologists are sometimes confronted with the unpleasant task of informing clients and family members of assessment results that are difficult to share because the information is unwelcome. For example; presenting audiometric results that confirm the suspected profound hearing loss of a two-year-old, explaining the results of a receptive language test that place a developmentally delayed four-year-old below the first percentile, sharing the cognitive assessment results with a family following their twenty-year-old son's severe head trauma, and explaining to adult children that their beloved mother's global aphasia may be irreversible, are situations that are not unfamiliar to clinicians. In other instances, the clinician is sure that small changes in family interaction will benefit the client, but family members seem unable to make these changes (see Chapter 12 for a discussion of this situation).The counseling techniques as well as knowledge of the grieving process make it possible for us to address these concerns in a helpful way.

Responding to Expressions of Emotion

Communicative disorders naturally create an array of feelings that may be expressed by the client and/or family members. These feelings can be different for each family member, and if the disorder is associated with a permanent disability, will emerge, disappear, and re-emerge throughout the family life cycle. Expression of these feelings is a normal part of the adaptation to the problem and should be viewed as natural and acceptable by the clinician. When the clinician or other professionals associated with the client and family attempt to ignore and or disqualify these feelings (e.g., "Don't be upset, we'll get some hearing aids on Johnny, and then we can teach him to talk"), the family's *normal* grief process may be subverted in a way that will be detrimental to treatment. We call this "professional denial" since the clinician may be pretending that the situation is not as grievous as it is in order to avoid the emotions associated with the problem.

Honest expression of feelings must be acknowledged and supported in order for families to engage in the serious work of treatment. Further, referral to a psychologist or counselor may compound the problem in some cases. Family members who had been referred for counseling by other professionals have told us of thinking, "Now, in addition to all I am going through, I have been referred to *another* counselor. There must be something really wrong with me." Most families do not need additional psychological counseling when the clinician is able to accept and respond appropriately to tears, anger, depression, and other *normal* expressions of feeling. The calm presence of an empathic clinician who uses reflection and neutral questioning will benefit clients and family members as they express the emotions created by the circumstances associated with a communicative disorder.

Communicating With Co-Workers, Supervisors and Supervisees

Speech-language pathologists and audiologists work together in many capacities as students, professors, supervisors, and members of treatment teams. A common interest in learning about and treating communicative disorders unites them in their work. Nevertheless, differences sometimes emerge and problem solving is desirable as these differences are assessed and solutions are developed. When at least one member of the dyad or group in question is able to use counseling techniques, problems can be identified and solved with greater ease than when these skills are not accessed.

Communicating With Professionals From Different Treatment Orientations

Many speech-language pathologists and audiologists are members of treatment teams composed of professionals with varying professional backgrounds relative to communicatively disordered persons and their families. Each member of this professional system is concerned about the wellbeing of her clients and has a different perspective of treatment. The use of counseling techniques will help the speech-language pathologist maintain a polyocular view, assess the resources that are available, and cooperate in developing effective treatment plans. We believe, of course, that the clients' family members should also be equal partners in this treatment planning.

USING THE TECHNIQUES

The techniques described here are used by family therapists, speech-language pathologists, children, parents, spouses, counselors, psychologists, teachers, business people, grandparents and all manner of human beings who want to interact successfully with clients, family members and co-workers. These techniques have usually been identified, described and taught by counseling professionals but are not owned by them and may be used by any person who finds pleasure in initiating creative change-producing human contact. We will describe these techniques as we use them and encourage the reader to be adventurous and creative in adapting them to her own personal style.

Joining

The speech-language pathologist gains acceptance of and admittance into the family system through the process of joining (Minuchin, 1974). This is accomplished by acknowledging and promoting the family's strengths, respecting the established roles of family members, and by affirming the self-worth of each individual (Simon, et al., 1985). As the joining process evolves, family members begin to know that the clinician understands and respects each person's point of view. This accommodation to the family's perspective promotes a willingness on the part of family members to hear and understand the clinician's professional ideas regarding treatment. Joining becomes a reciprocally beneficial process, and a new interactive system is formed, one that includes all members as equal partners on the treatment team (see Chapter 2).

The joining process begins with the first telephone or in-person contact and continues into the first and subsequent family meetings. Most professionals experience a sense of excitement, some trepidation, and genuine interest in wanting to get to know a new family group. As the first meeting begins, the clinician listens respectfully, responds nonjudgmentally, and begins to experience the concerns, struggles, satisfactions, and hopes that the family members bring to the session. The clinician also begins to understand the family members' views of reality (Minuchin, 1974). An early sign that the joining process is underway occurs when the family members show interest in continuing to work with the clinician. As treatment continues, the family and clinician interact in an increasingly cooperative manner. A trusting alliance is formed that facilitates joint decision-making and positive change in the family environment of the person with a communicative disorder. Gradually, a bond is established that assures the family's involved participation in the habilitation process.

Behaviors that may be adopted to facilitate the joining process are the following: socializing about everyday issues, mirroring the posture of the person being listened to, using language and terminology that matches the family's level of understanding, matching family members' affect (smiling, frowning, looking puzzled), and identifying each family member's unique interests and attributes. Most of these behaviors evolve quite naturally when the professional is committed to an appreciation of the family members' and client's points of view.

Attending

Attending is conveyed through posturing and is a part of the listening and clarifying process (Rogers, 1965). In order to attend fully to each member of the family, the clinician positions him/herself so that eye contact is possible with each family member. Chairs should be arranged, for example, in a circle. Toys, manuals, and other equipment should be placed on a side table next to the clinician. Attention to each person's verbal and non-verbal communication is shown through cues such as eye contact, nodding of the head, naturally friendly facial expressions, and an open-body position. A strong desire to understand each person's thoughts, feelings, hopes, and fears regarding the communicative problem should be experienced by the clinician. This desire tends to be conveyed to the family and, in turn, helps family members relax. Family members and clients invariably respond positively to an attentive, concerned professional.

Listening

"Someone who really listens to me" is at the top of the list of characteristics that speech-language clinicians identify when asked who they like to talk to when they have something important to say. When Gehart-Brooks & Lyle (1999) asked psychotherapy clients about change and what was helpful in therapy, "all clients identified therapist listening as most significant" (p. 25). When we ask the parents of our clients what they like most about their child's clinician they often respond, "He listened to my ideas and concerns." The clinician is assured of developing a good relationship with the parents of his clients if he listens respectfully to them. This skill can be difficult to develop as we live in a culture that values speaking over listening. Clarification and reflection are two techniques that can be used to hone listening skills.

Clarification

The content and communicative intent of the speaker's verbal and nonverbal expressions become clear as the clinician attends to each family member, accepts silence to allow the speaker an opportunity to think about responses, nods and utters an occasional "mm-hm," and restates what the speaker has said. Each of these responses conveys to the speaker, "I am listening to you very carefully" (Benjamin, 1981).

Clarification is the interviewer's restatement for the interviewee of what the latter has said or tried to say (Benjamin. 1981). The response may be simplified to make it clearer and more understandable, but the meaning and intent expressed by the speaker should always be maintained. The goal is to develop a clear understanding of the speaker's perspective while also helping the speaker to clarify his/her own ideas. Clarification encourages the speaker to continue and also promotes the joining process. The following is an example of clarification as it was used with a family that was concerned about their two and one-half-year-old child with a language delay.

Father: Whenever I try to get Chris to talk to me, he just doesn't say anything. . . . ummm. . . Carol (his wife, who is also present) can at least get him to make some kind of, uh, sound or use motions with his hands.

Clinician: You've really tried hard to get Chris to talk. . .but. . .just haven't had much luck with that.

Father: Yeh, I don't know if he doesn't hear me or. . . . if he's just stubborn, or maybe I'm talking to him wrong, or something. . . . .

Clinician: It sounds like you've thought of lots of possibilities, and . . you'd really like to know why Chris isn't more responsive.

Father: Yeah, we came here today because we thought you could help with that. What do you think is wrong?

Clinician: (responding directly to the father's question, discontinuing clarification) Well . . . that's a good question. Right now, I don't know, but as we work together and learn more about what you and Carol have noticed. . . and as we do a speech-language assessment. . . I think we should be able to find some beginning answers.

Useful information was gleaned from this brief bit of clarification. The clinician learned that the father is concerned, has tried unsuccessfully to elicit speech and language, and is seeking help from an "expert." The clinician indicated that she understood his perspective, used language of participation, joined him in his quest for "answers," and reiterated that the parents and clinician would operate as a team as the language delay is assessed and treated. At this early stage, care was taken to resist becoming the "answer person." Instead, the clinician indicated that further exploration of the problem was necessary.

Clarification is a useful interviewing skill because family members will let the clinician know if she has missed the intent of what is being said, thus offering opportunity to restate in a different way. For example, imagine resuming the clarification sequence during the second interchange. Notice that the interchange takes a different twist as the father corrects a clarification statement that was not quite on target.

Clinician: It sounds like you've thought of lots of possibilities, and . . you'd really like to know why Chris isn't more responsive.

Father: Well no, I. . uh. . . really don't have any idea about what the problem could be. I don't care what's causing this thing with Chris, I just want to do something about it.

Clinician: O.K., the causes aren't important to you, but you're eager to get some treatment started.

Father: Yeah, he's already three years old and should be talking by now. I just want to know what we can do!

Clinician: (responding directly to the father's statement, discontinuing clarification) Good, I want to get Carol's ideas now, then do a speech-language assessment, and then we'll figure out something that we can all do to help Chris communicate better.

A different initial understanding has been gathered from the changed interaction between the father and the clinician. The first exchange indicated a desire for "answers" and the second a desire for "action." This understanding of the father's perspective will help the clinician strategize for change and design an appropriate assignment. Another important benefit that has been derived from either exchange is that the father has begun to sense that he is dealing with a professional that respects his opinions and is willing to accommodate his concerns for his son.

Reflection

Reflection, a skill described by Carl Rogers (Rogers, 1965), is similar to clarification but also includes the restatement of feelings in order to help the individual access the deeper meanings being expressed. Roger's model proposes that when this technique is used by a congruent professional, who demonstrates unconditional positive regard, individuals are able to sort out and solve vexing problems using their own personal resources. Many of the problems that families must face when their member has a communicative disorder do not have clear-cut solutions. Furthermore, when professionals tell family members how they *should* feel (e.g. "Don't feel bad, everything will be O.K," or, "You shouldn't be saying things like that; it will make Sarah feel worse") feelings are denied and potential personal resources are buried within the individual. Instead, when the speech-language pathologist responds to expressions of feelings, the joining process is enhanced and family members are given permission to deal with the frustration, pain and confusion that they are experiencing. This participation promotes a sense of trust between the family members and clinician.

The clinician can use reflection when strong feelings are being expressed and/or when the feeling content of the speaker's statements is evident. When the family is experiencing a crisis associated with a communicative handicap such as might occur with diagnosis of hearing loss, autism, a serious head trauma, the birth of a child with a cleft lip, or a stroke resulting in aphasia, feelings are often evident. Strong feelings also may be expressed as family members show anger, disappointment, sorrow, happiness, confusion, exhaustion, etc. related to difficulties that may seem less serious to the professional. When the communicative disorder is associated with a permanent disability, these feelings, particularly anger, may appear to be directed at the clinician. Usually these feelings are directed at the unfairness of the disability itself and at the family's perplexing and painful situation. Understanding this will help the professional respond appropriately with reflective listening.

Some clinicians are comfortable with expressions of feelings and use reflection during the first family meeting even if it is not a crisis situation. The success of this technique, early in treatment, depends upon the clinician's intent. If the intent is to show respect and understanding and to clearly reflect what is being said, even when this is different from what the clinician thinks should be said or felt, the technique is likely to enhance the clinician-family partnership. The clinician's decision to use reflection will depend upon the strength of the emotions being expressed and his personal comfort with the technique. As with clarification, the speaker will correct the clinician if the reflection is off-target but will continue to express him/herself knowing that an effort is being made to understand the feelings and ideas being shared. Our experience has been that a few reflective statements help release the emotional pain being expressed. Family members let us know when they are ready to continue efforts directed toward speech-language change, knowing that the clinician understands their need to deal with these feelings at the same time that work continues.

The following excerpt continues the interview begun earlier and shows the use of reflective listening during a first session:

Clinician: Carol, John's noticed that you can get Chris to talk to you and to use motions from time to time. Can you tell me more about this?

Mother: Well. . . . . . I suppose he does use more sounds when he's with me, but I get so tired of trying to get him to say something and sometimes just get mad because I think he *could* do a lot more than he tries to do, and I don't like it when he uses motions because I think that's just an excuse not to talk.

Clinician: It sounds like you get pretty upset and. . maybe . . feel like giving up sometimes because Chris doesn't want to try to talk to you.

Mother: Yeah. . . . . He's really not a bad kid, but it's so hard to know what he wants when he starts to holler, or turns away from me, or gives up trying. I. . . . I . . . don't think he means to be so stubborn because sometimes he starts to cry when I get upset with him, and then he hangs on me like he's afraid I'm going to leave him or something like that. I'm almost at my wits end with all of this.

Clinician: Mm. . .hm. . .this problem is bothering you a lot and you'd really like to figure out how to get Chris to *try* to respond to you so you two could maybe enjoy each other a little bit. . . . . instead of always feeling so frustrated.

Mother: Oh, yeah. . . . . that would sure be nice, but I don't have a clue about how to get it to happen.

Clinician: O.K. . . . . .this whole thing has been tough for you, and John (husband) and you both want to figure out what can be done to motivate Chris to talk more. I'd like to ask a few more questions about what you two have noticed, and then we'll move on to figuring our what we can *do*. Does that seem O.K. with you?

Mother: Sure, I'll try *anything* to get him talking.

The use of reflection helped Chris's mother express her frustration and also let her know that the clinician was comfortable with the feeling statements that are a natural part of a family's response to a communicative disorder. Incidentally, more data were gathered about the mother's interactive responses to Chris's language delay. Since many of their interchanges ended in conflict, and this was frustrating to both of them, it was learned that Chris's mother would like to experience a decrease in this kind of interaction. Again, reflection was discontinued when mother seemed, in this communicative interchange, to be finished expressing her feelings. The clinician, however, continued to indicate that solving the problem required a joint effort, and that the family's thoughts and ideas were respected and important.

Not all family members express feelings, and not all clinicians are able to respond reflectively to family members who do express deeper emotions. Nevertheless, reflection is a useful skill to cultivate since its occasional use will open the interactive treatment process to greater understanding, empathy, and change. Reflection, clarification, and questioning are not mutually exclusive activities. These interconnected skills are used to move the treatment process in the direction of cooperative efforts aimed at establishing clear goals and procedures relative to speech-language change.

Questioning

Open questions elicit more information than closed questions. A closed question can only be answered with a yes, no, or a short phrase. Some closed questions *must* be asked such as the following: What is Justin's birthdate?; What is your physician's name?; Have you met with other professionals to discuss the communicative problem?; etc. Once these essential closed questions have been asked, the clinician should shift to asking open questions. Open questions give the client or family member an opportunity to respond in a variety of ways. For example, instead of asking, "Do you like to play with Nathan?" (closed question); ask, "What do you enjoy doing with Nathan?" (open question). Instead of asking, "How often where you fluent last week?" (closed question); say, "Tell me about the times when were you most fluent last week." (open question). Open questions enrich the flow of the clinical conversation.

The *intent* of the questioner also influences the effect of questions. Questions asked from a position of neutrality (Fleuridas, et al., 1986; Tomm, 1988) are more useful than questions that are intended to teach or upbraid. The clinician will operate from a position of neutrality if he is genuinely interested, respectful and curious as he gathers new information. We like to adopt an ethnographic stance as this helps us ask questions from a position of neutrality. Our intent, then, is exploratory, and our questions are asked with an intense desire to learn how the family members think about and respond to issues associated with the communicative disorder.

Questions must be intermingled with clarification and reflection. When the client or family member responds to a question, clarification helps the clinician fully understand the response and use this understanding to inform the next question. Good questions are always reflexive (Tomm, 1988). This means that each question is a response to the client's last response which has been carefully clarified. The questioning process can be compared to a tennis match. Each tennis player knows how he'll return the ball only after the opponent's ball has landed in his court. In like manner, each question asked during an interview is determined by the response (where the ball has landed in the clinician's court) of the family member to the clinician's last question. Open, neutral, reflexive questions used in tandem with clarification and reflection contribute to an interesting, informative interview.

Summarizing

Summarizing helps the clinician remember what has been learned, elicits more information and provides closure at transition points. For example, when the family interview portion of the first session is completed, the clinician should summarize what has been said. "You, John, want to *do* something about Chris's talking problem. Carol, you're sometimes at your wits end and get pretty discouraged but still have enough energy to try something else. You're both eager to learn how to help Chris communicate better and hope that I will be able to offer ideas that will help. Does this sum up what you've told me so far?" When the family indicates that the summary statement is accurate, the clinician is ready to move to the next phase of the session. In this case the summary statement provides a natural link to the clinical evaluation.

The clinician should be careful to use language that matches the family's language level, and the summary must show sensitivity to their view of the problem. The anticipation and act of summarizing helps the clinician organize and remember important data related to the family's perspective of the speech-language problem. It also informs his thinking about the upcoming clinical evaluation as he will pay special attention to the areas of concern raised by family members.

Solution-Focused Tracking

Tracking is a technique described by Minuchin (1974) who uses it as part of the joining process to help the family and clinician develop an understanding of the family's structure. Our use of tracking focuses on identifying family resources rather than family structure. We track a family's interactive patterns in two ways. First, by asking neutral questions and then using clarifying statements in response to these questions, we learn about family responses to communicative events as these occur in sequences of behavior. As we attend to the family members' descriptions of interactive events, communicative sequences are identified, and new information about the contextual issues surrounding the problem are discovered. Second, we observe family interaction as it spontaneously occurs in the session, or we request an enactment (Minuchin, 1974) in order to observe in-session interaction relating to the communicative disorder. We do this from a solution-focused perspective by paying attention to strengths rather than deficits. Once we have a clear understanding of the speech-language problem, we begin tracking exceptions to the problem. In other words, we're interested in learning about what the family does that works rather than what they do that doesn't work.

Solution-focused tracking usually creates systemic thinking that is new to both the family and the clinician. Ideas about how to build change into the family system begin to evolve as family members and clinician alike gain new insights into the situation. A family member's response to each question influences the clinician's clarification of the response and the formation of the next question. Each interview is a unique, idiosyncratic event created and shaped by the clinician's responses to family members and provides a rich array of data to be used in strategizing for change.

The following excerpt shows how questions asked from a neutral position facilitate the solution-focused tracking process:

Clinician: Carol, you said that there are many times when you try to help Chris talk. Let's talk about what happened the last time you did that. (open, neutral request)

Mother: Well . . . . it's hard to remember an exact time. . . . . .

Father: . . . . what about when you're in the kitchen trying to get something cooked and he's in there fussing and carrying on, and you can't figure out what he's saying?

Mother: Yeah . . . . that seems to happen every day . . . and . . . yeah, that happened last night. I was really in a hurry because I'd just gotten home from work and, John, you were trying to clean up the house, and Chris was fussy . . . . seems like he's usually fussy at night . . . and he was trying to tell me something, I think, but I couldn't figure it out at all.

Clinician: O.K . . this is a good everyday example . . . that's what we want to look at. So . . . you're in the kitchen trying to fix something to eat, and John's cleaning up the house . . . . (clarification)

Mother: . . . . . Yeah . . . . and don't forget Samantha's (ten-month-old daughter) also fussing because she's hungry too.

Clinician: O.K . . things are pretty hectic for everyone right then and in the midst of all this Chris is wanting to communicate something, and you can't figure it out at all. What do you do? (clarification/neutral question)

Mother: Well, I usually stop what I'm doing and look at him and say, "Tell me again; I can't understand you!"

Clinician: What happens then? (tracking interactive pattern)

Mother: He makes those sounds again, and I keep trying to figure it out.

Clinician: You really want to know what he's saying. How do you respond? (clarification/neutral question/tracking interactive pattern)

Mother: Well . . . . sometimes I can tell what he's trying to say because he's pointing at something, usually some kind of food, so I might say, "cracker, is that what you want, a cracker?"

Clinician: When you ask him if he wants a cracker, as he's pointing in the direction of the crackers, how does he respond? (neutral question/tracking interactive pattern)

Mother: Well . . . . if I've guessed right, he nods his head and then I usually give him a cracker and he's happy for a few minutes. If I guessed wrong, he hollers louder, and I keep on trying to figure out what he's trying to say. After two or three guesses, I give up and he starts crying and runs to John, and John starts to play with him or something like that.

Clinician: So when Chris is trying to tell you something and you can figure it out from his motions and sounds, he's happy for a little while. If you can't figure it out, he keeps trying and sometimes cries, and if John's around, runs to him. (clarification/ tracking interactive pattern/ resources identified)

Mother: Uh huh . . . . that's about it.

Clinician: John, is this about how you see it happening too? (neutral question/tracking father's response)

Father: Yep, except I don't even try to figure out what he's saying because it's impossible for me.

Clinician: What do you do instead? (solution-focused tracking question)

Father: Usually, I'll try to play with him or something so he'll quiet down so Carol can finish cooking because I'm pretty hungry by then! (John and Carol both laugh at John's joke, look at each other and smile as they share their mutual frustration).

This brief tracking excerpt elicited a great deal of helpful information. Chris appears to have a clear desire to communicate with his mother, Carol, but is unable to do so in a manner that is rewarding to the two of them. Carol has the ability to figure out Chris's meaning even when under considerable stress. His father, John, is willing to help out when things become hectic relative to Chris's behavior. In addition, the nonverbal alliance shown by Chris's parents indicated that they support one another during the stressful times associated with normal daily living. Although additional tracking and the speech-language assessment are yet to occur, the clinician can begin to formulate a hypothesis about this particular family's resources and can fit those resources to an appropriate first step relative to speech-language change.

Tracking is *not* done to figure out what is wrong with the family. It is done to uncover interactive resources, particularly those that can be accessed for change and then used to treat the communicative disorder. This example shows a determined and resourceful child, a creative mother who can "figure things out," and a father willing to be supportive and wanting to "do something." Carol and John seem to enjoy a friendly relationship despite their difficulties and show an ability to cooperate with one another and with the clinician. These resources will be very useful as the clinician and family continue their quest for change.

A second kind of solution-focused tracking occurs when family members enact spontaneous examples of interactive events. For example, when an adult daughter begins to communicate with her aphasic mother, a brother plays with his language-delayed sister, or a father discusses a problem with his head-injured teenager, the clinician will want to observe this behavior to identify family resources that can be used to help the person with the communicative disorder. If spontaneous events do not occur, the clinician can ask family members to discuss an issue, read a book to a child, play a game with an adolescent, etc., making certain that the activity is within the framework of the family's ability and understanding. We often request enactments in follow-up sessions as a way of observing the family's integration of new behaviors into their natural style. Usually, during early sessions, the family is more comfortable showing spontaneous interactions. The clinician's job is to allow these to take place without interfering.

Tracking helps the clinician gather data about the interactive patterns in which the communicative disorder is embedded. These data are "stored" in the clinician's mental file of information and will be used to appropriately link the family's idiosyncratic style to desired speech-language changes. As the treatment process evolves, attention is paid to the useful resources that are uncovered since these must be reinforced and appreciated. The clinician may also notice behaviors that may be reinforcing the persistence of the problem, but those will be intentionally ignored as positive behaviors are discovered, strengthened, and reinforced. The solution-focused tracking process also helps family members themselves uncover attributes and ideas that lead to changed behaviors. As they think about the interactive events related to their family member's communicative disorder in new and different ways, they tend to acquire insights heretofore unexplored.

Creative Strategizing

As the family session continues, the clinician and family develop an understanding of the problem as it is experienced in the natural context. They are joined in their desire for positive change; patterns of interaction in which the problem is embedded have been identified; and clinical testing has occurred (see Chapter 3). The clinician-client-family team must now use this information to create change.

Creative strategizing, the process that initiates this change, has been adapted from the work of strategic family therapists (Haley, 1976; Madanes, 1981). "Strategic therapists set clear goals which always include solving the presenting problem. The emphasis is not on a method to be applied to all cases but on designing a strategy for each specific problem. Since the therapy focuses on the social context of human dilemmas, the therapist's task is to design an intervention in the client's social situation" (Madanes, 1981, p.19). Creative strategizing, as we use it, begins as the clinician starts to formulate hypotheses about the family's interactive resources and connects these strengths to desired speech-language change. Creative strategizing culminates in a simple, yet effective assignment that is discussed and, if necessary, refined with the family's input.

The speech-language pathologist begins the creative strategizing process at the time of the first family contact and continues to think about strategies for change as information is gathered and summarized. Strategizing focuses on creating task assignments that will facilitate speech-language change. Care is taken to design assignments that encourage family members to maintain their established roles while respecting their view of reality. Creative strategizing "flavors" the entire treatment process and is the result of joining the clinician's expertise with the family's idiosyncratic style in a continuously evolving manner. The therapeutic system is nudged in the direction of positive speech-language change through the goals and procedures that are outlined and discussed at each session (see Chapter 6).

Assigning Tasks

According to Haley (1976), there are three purposes to assigning tasks. These are to encourage people to behave differently, to intensify the relationship with the therapist, and to gather information. With this in mind, the outcome of a task assignment is never considered a failure. Careful tracking of behavior surrounding attempts to implement an assignment provides the clinician and family with new data regarding the communicative disorder and informs the creative strategizing process so that new assignments may be developed. Two skills aid us in assigning tasks: the use of a compliment and an egalitarian assignment delivery.

First, we find that the use of a compliment is an excellent prelude to the delivery of the task. deShazer (1985) and his team of family therapists describe the therapeutic use of the compliment and make it a powerful part of their model for family and individual change. The speech-language pathologist's compliment may be directed to the family as a whole or to individual family members and should always be based on information gathered during the family interview portion of the session. Compliments may be general such as, "We are very impressed by your willingness to find a time when all of you could meet to help us figure out how best to help your mother. Your concern for her is clearly evident" (delivered to the adult children and their spouses of a 78-year-old woman with global aphasia). Or, the compliment can be specific to family members. For example, "Sean (eight-year-old brother of language delayed four-year-old female), we noticed that you played with Jennifer very nicely tonight. You listened to everything she said and even repeated some of the words she used to show her that you understood her. That was very good! . . . . . Sheila (mother), your expansion of Jennifer's sentences is impressive. When Jennifer says, 'cookie gone', you respond with, 'The cookie's gone, the cookie's all gone.' That's excellent. We think her progress is related to your remembering to do this . . . . Jim (father), you continue to play with Jennifer in an attentive, calm way . . . . . this helps her attend to the activity at hand as well as to your talking together. Keep up the good work. Now, let's think about adding something new to our efforts. This week we suggest you try to _____ " The clinician can also write a brief compliment on the family's assignment sheet.

With the eventual delivery of a compliment in mind, the professional "tunes in" to the family's resources, and this effort becomes part of the creative strategizing process. The compliment also paves the way for the family's acceptance of the assignment which, of course, is designed to fit their ability to cooperate in the treatment process. The compliment also helps the family become more comfortable with their role on the treatment team. Unfortunately, many families seem to expect criticism and informal lectures about what they are doing wrong. When this does not happen, and an honest compliment is delivered instead, they become empowered to participate in a more cooperative and active manner. The compliment is derived from the clinician's honest appraisal of the family's resources and should never be phony. With some families, compliments are easy to give, and one can readily choose from several options. With other families a concerted effort must be made to find appropriate compliments, but one can usually be found.

Second, (as described in Chapter 5) the task must be carefully linked to the family's resources and should be delivered in an egalitarian manner. The task assignment may be prefaced with phrases such as, "How about trying _____"; "Since it seemed to help Sarah when I did_____ , what do you think of your trying _____?"; I wonder what you think of this idea. . . . . . . ?" This kind of delivery demonstrates equality and continues to emphasize the importance of a cooperative relationship between the clinician and the family. When the assignment is framed in an egalitarian way and is carefully designed to connect family resources to the desired speech-language changes, it is almost always accepted. Modifications and changes suggested by the family are welcomed, and these are used to make the assignment more closely "fit" their ability to cooperate.

Use of Self

The clinician's personal reactions to his work with families are a rich source of data. His emotional responses and personal ideas offer clues about the family's processes as well as his involvement in them. A clinician's feelings of failure when a child with autism doesn't respond to carefully crafted assignments, a clinician's sadness when he must tell parents that their toddler has a profound hearing loss, a clinician's disappointment when a family fails to attend a scheduled appointment, can all be used to facilitate the speech-language treatment process.

Use of self begins with the clinician respecting and acknowledging his personal reactions. These reactions should be accepted nonjudgmentally since they are a natural part of professional life. Once the reaction is recognized, the clinician should decide what to do with it. Sometimes this decision must be made quickly as a response could be immediately useful. Every response should be preceded by the clinician asking himself, "Will my response to my reaction be beneficial to my client and the family?" If the answer is "no," comment should be withheld. If the answer is "yes," the clinician can acknowledge his feelings in one of several ways.

First, he can decide to withhold comment because the time is not right. For example, he has informed parents at an initial meeting that their toddler is profoundly deaf. The parents react with shock, and the child's mother begins to cry. The clinician feels tears welling in his eyes and wonders what he should do with his personal feelings of sadness. He decides that these young parents need to be in the presence of a composed, empathic, caring clinician who will not "fall apart." He swallows his sadness, decides to share his reactions with a colleague after the session, and begins to reflect the parent's grief. At another time, with another family that he has been working with for some time, he may decide that sharing his sadness is an appropriate response.

Second, he can plug his reaction back into the family system. If, for example, he is feeling a sense of failure because a child with autism isn't responding to his well-planned interventions, he may hypothesize that family members have similar feelings and say, "You must feel discouraged after doing so many things to help Ryan and seeing so little change." The clinician's personal reactions can be helpful when reflecting the family's current feelings.

Third, he can use an I-statement. An I-statement begins with "I", describes a feeling about a situation, and may request a change. For example, the clinician recognizes that he is disappointed because a family failed to keep an appointment. He may decide to call them and say, "I was really disappointed when you weren't able to make it to our session. I hope everything is OK and would like to ask that in the future you give me a call if you are unable to attend." Most people can hear and respect an I-statement more easily than a "you" statement or an attempt to act pleasant when the clinician is really quite annoyed.

Clinician's should practice listening to themselves, respecting their personal reactions and then using these to make decisions about their clinical work. A congruent, honest clinician who is fully present and available to his clients will be respected by them and by their family members. Further, the clinician will avoid the stress that is often associated with repressed feelings.

UNDERSTANDING THE GRIEVING AND LOSS PROCESS

Families with a member who has a communicative disorder often experience grief as an emerging, disappearing, re-emerging, disappearing, re-emerging etc. process. According to Moses (1985), "You – the special educator, audiologist, speech-language pathologist – are the ones who deal firsthand with people who are under stress in a circumstance that is most appropriately dealt with by you rather than by psychologists, social workers, or psychiatrists. You are the people who can take a truly holistic approach in the treatment of the child within a nonpathology-oriented environment" (p. 84). We agree with this perspective and add to it our belief that this is true for clients and family members at every stage of the family life cycle, not just for families with children. When the professional uses reflective listening and responds to expressions of feeling as they occur, this normalizes the grieving and loss process and gives family members permission to be honest about their feelings and thoughts. When the clinician becomes frightened by these expressions and immediately refers to another professional because he is uncomfortable, this creates another problem for the family. Family members may think that there is now something else wrong with them, thereby adding to the stress they are already experiencing. In most cases when family members decide to seek professional counseling, this will be a choice that they themselves initiate. The clinician should strongly support their decision. The clinician's willingness to allow expressions of feeling helps those who want additional counseling to be empowered to seek that help when they have decided that they are ready. We rarely have experienced a need to refer to a family therapist, psychologist, social worker, or psychiatrist for counseling but would not hesitate to do so if we were certain that it was in the best interest of our clients. Once the referral is made, it is up to the client and family to decide if they want to act on the suggestion that has been offered.

Stages of Loss

Several authors have described stages of crisis and loss by suggesting process models to consider when dealing with the emotions expressed by clients and family members who are dealing with issues of disability (Fortier and Wanlass, 1984; Moses, 1985; Spanbock, 1987). The crisis stages suggested by Fortier and Wanlass (1984) will be used here, acknowledging that other models can be equally helpful. The clinician should be familiar with crisis stages so that he can respond appropriately to family members. Therefore, counseling responses are described as well. The stages are impact, denial, grief, focusing outward, and closure (Fortier and Wanlass, 1984).

Impact occurs when the family and client first learn of the disability or of an accident that is likely to lead to future disability. An infant born with a bilateral cleft lip and palate, diagnosis of severe to profound hearing loss, a closed head injury, or a stroke are examples of events that trigger the impact stage. When the communicative disorder is one of the results of a life-threatening accident, there may be a brief period of elation related to the relief of knowing that the loved one will not die (Spanbock, 1987). However, this elation is short-lived as reality sets in.

Sometimes, a family has suspected that something is wrong for several weeks, months, or years, and the agonizing wait finally culminates in a diagnosis that confirms their fears. This may occur when a hearing loss is diagnosed, an infant's cerebral palsy is identified, or the effects of a head injury become clearly evident. In these cases the impact stage may be prolonged, but a point is always reached where the reality of the situation impacts the family and the client. During the impact stage family members experience numbness, disorientation, nausea, agitation, muscle tension, and a number of other physically and emotionally destabilizing effects. This is certainly not a time for professional lectures or cheerful assurances that "everything is going to be just fine." Instead, the professional should present all information in its simplest form, knowing that the same information will probably have to be repeated later since not all of it will be "heard." Questions should be answered honestly, directly and simply. The clinician should allow silence and give family members an opportunity to say what they need to say. The clinician can use reflection as needed and show a calm presence that offers assurance of future assistance even as the family and client are grieving their loss.

The *denial* stage may begin soon after impact or may emerge weeks or months later. Moses (1985) reiterates that denial is necessary, healthy, and important and buys time for people to find the inner strength and the external supports to deal with the "undealable." Luterman (1984), also confirms that " . . . denial is a very normal and human reaction, which occurs in all of us" (p.150). The wise clinician will view family denial in this same way. Furthermore, it is advisable to avoid "professional denial" that occurs when the clinician pretends that nothing tragic has happened and that the disability can be fully overcome. During the denial stage, family members may experience tenseness, anxiety, ambivalence, disbelief, anger, avoidance, and may "shop" for cures. The clinician can use clarification, reflection and neutral questioning as the family and client struggle to figure out which issues that they can and cannot handle. Family members can work on plans for change even while the denial is present. The clinician's understanding of this will be woven into the fabric of treatment.

Grief is another stage in the loss process that may also overlap the previous two stages. Grief is often expressed through crying. Anger, withdrawal, sleeplessness, guilt, self-doubt, questioning and reliving the past are other common expressions associated with this stage. Again, the professional should exhibit a calm presence and allow these expressions of feeling to occur. Reflection should be used to acknowledge feelings. As this is done, most family members will dry their tears, at least temporarily, and ask to continue with the treatment process.

Focusing outward is the stage that evolves out of the previous three. Family members express relief that "the worst is over," show renewed energy and confidence, become active in considering options, and seek new knowledge and information. Other expressions of feeling may reappear during this stage, but the general tone is one of hope and fresh optimism.

Persons who have been free to express the feelings felt during the impact, denial, and grief stages are likely to enter this phase with a sense of renewal in spite of the monumental challenges that lie ahead. Clarification, neutral questioning, creative strategizing, and task assignment can all be utilized by the clinician during the focusing outward stage.

Fortier and Wanlass' (1984) last stage is *closure*. At this time family members are generally calm and relaxed and have adjusted to their changed family member. The physical symptoms experienced earlier will have diminished considerably. Family members often say, "I'm able to sleep again," or, "I can finally enjoy eating again." Continuing external support, creative strategizing, clarification, neutral questioning, and task assignment are techniques that should be used as treatment efforts proceed, sometimes on a long-term basis.

Variations in the Loss Process

The professional's understanding of the loss process will increase his sensitivity to the emotional and physical pain that often accompanies speech-language disorders. Counseling responses can be woven into the fabric of treatment in a way that may seem almost imperceptible to someone unfamiliar with the power of respectful and empathic listening. The stages and counseling responses are described here to give the clinician techniques to use when the need arises. These do not supplant the clinician's primary task which is to involve the family in the treatment process. Nevertheless, additional consideration must be given to the following factors since these also relate to the grieving and loss process.

Every individual in a family will respond differently to the loss experienced and is likely to traverse the stages with different pacing and timing. For example, a father may show little emotion especially during the early phases of the process, perhaps because he desires to remain strong in light of his wife's open expression of grief, or he may be a person who usually does not show emotion, and this becomes a time when that particular personality trait is evident. Conversely, he may be very open to showing disappointment, sorrow and anger while his partner evidences little overt expression of feelings. An individual whose life pattern has been to accept disappointment in a calm manner will continue to show that same pattern as the current distress is felt. An individual whose style is to openly express feelings will continue to respond overtly when grief and loss are experienced. Respect for these individual differences is necessary, and the professional is advised to refrain from "telling" people what they *should* be feeling or which stage they *should* be experiencing. The loss stages are offered as a guide for professionals who want to be sensitive to the grieving process while also respectful of individual and family differences. A polyocular perspective will aid in the successful treatment of families that are experiencing and expressing grief.

The grief process is not one that is smoothly traversed and then completed. Stages repeat themselves, sorrow and pain may re-emerge at developmental transitions, and "mini" grief processes may appear for a few hours, days, or even years after the original impact has occurred. One father told us that he had forgotten that his son Carl was developmentally disabled until he enrolled him in preschool and saw the other children attending the special class. At that time he was once again reminded that Carl was not "normal." This father had evolved through the loss process to closure over a period of thirteen to fourteen months as he and his wife worked together to provide for and enjoy their son. As Carl approached and began his developmental transition into the preschool years, elements of the loss process re-emerged, and the parents experienced several days of renewed grief that was, however, not as intense as it had been during the early stages of the loss process. These feelings are likely to re-emerge when Carl starts elementary school, when his age cohorts begin dating and driving, when the time for adult independence arrives, and as his parents age and become concerned about his lifetime care.

Finally, the loss process is experienced at every phase of the family life cycle. An aging couple whose retirement plans are changed by a debilitating stroke, a young adult whose life plans are wiped out by a severe head injury, and a young family giving up their dream of a "perfect" child all need the skills of a sensitive clinician as they and other family members work to solve the speech-language problems that are a significant part of their loss.

SUMMARY

Counseling techniques enhance the effectiveness of the speech-language clinician during all phases of Family-Based Treatment. Like the fresh basil in a fine tomato sauce, the blue thread in a woven fabric, or the second violin in a string orchestra, these techniques become an integral part of the process and outcome of treatment. Family-Based Treatment may be possible without their use but will be more satisfying, complete, and successful when these human relation skills are used by the clinician during the treatment process.

CHAPTER 9

APPLICATION TO EARLY INTERVENTION

One of the primary areas of change in speech-language pathology services during the past ten years has been in serving infants and toddlers and their families. Acronyms such as IFSP (Individualized Family Service Plan) and terms such as "family-centered" have become part of our profession's vocabulary. Even greater than the general expansion of services to a population, that were already being served to some extent, is the impact of the *manner* in which services to these infants and toddlers are to be delivered. Crais and Leonard (1990) expressed the concern of a profession in the title of their article, "99-457: Are Speech-Language Pathologists Ready for the Challenge?" The assumptions of the individual medical model are so pervasive and so consistently surround us in our professional literature, professional standards, conversations with colleagues, and professional conferences that it is very difficult to internalize "family-centered" thinking. In essence, that's what this book is all about; the Family-Based Treatment model is a model for providing family-centered services.

Family-Centered Treatment and Enabling Families

The definition of "family-centered" offered by Dunst, et al.(1991) has been accepted by nearly all who provide early intervention services. According to these authors, a family-centered approach is one in which families are in control of all decisions about their family member. The role of the speech-language pathologist, or other professional, is as a consultant to assist families as they make these decisions. Services are based upon strengths of families and are offered in such a manner that families are provided opportunities to demonstrate their strengths and abilities and develop new abilities.

Providing services in a manner that promotes positive changes in the child's speech-language and that, simultaneously, provide opportunities for families to show their strengths is referred to as "enabling" families (Donahue-Kilburg, 1992; McGonigel, et al., 1991). In order to do this, the early interventionist must provide an interactive environment in which these abilities and competencies may emerge. Four stragegies for creating such opportunities have been described (Andrews & Andrews, 1993). Among these strategies, and perhaps most useful, is encouraging all family members to participate in services. The clinician has more communicative resources with which to work when everyone is present. In our experience, the family's degree of comfort often is directly related to the number of family members present. In other words, it seems the more we are outnumbered, the freer family members are to encourage one another and to do something different. When family members are at ease, they are in a good position to demonstrate techniques they have used to help their child, participate in an assessment, interact with their child in a way that "introduces" the child to the clinician, and show the clinician strategies that they believe may potentially benefit their child. Of course, these activities benefit the joining process, too. When family members feel good about what they do, and the clinician has acknowledged their strengths, family members feel more confident and competent to help their toddler, and the clinician-family "fit" improves. The counseling techniques described in Chapter 8 provide the clinician with strategies for enabling family members. Joining, amplifying competencies, clarifying and reflecting, using neutral solution-focused questions, and developing isomorphic suggestions are among the techniques that promote enablement (Andrews & Andrews, 1993).

Families as Intergenerational Systems

It is generally agreed that a family systems framework provides the best basis for family-centered early intervention (Dunst, et al., 1991). An understanding of intergenerational influences, developmental family stages, developmental family tasks, transitional stressors, and developmental disruptions enhances the clinician's understanding and skill in using the Family-Based Treatment model, or any model of family-centered services. Families begin, evolve, change, and endure over a span of many years. As the life span increases, families expand to three, four, and sometimes five generations of individuals who are inextricably related through intergenerational time. Each generation moves through stages that evolve from one phase to another as members enter and leave the family system. Family theorists have suggested a number of different family developmental stage models (Duvall, 1977; Haley, 1973; Solomon, 1973). The model we use is one proposed by Carter and McGoldrick (1980). Their six-stage model begins with (1) the unattached young adult followed by (2) the joining of families through marriage. Subsequent family developmental stages include the following: (3) the family with young children; (4) the family with adolescents; (5) launching children and moving on; and (6) the family in later life. Developmental disruptions, such as divorce, remarriage, illness, early death, or disability have a profound effect on families as they evolve through these stages.

FAMILY DEVELOPMENTAL FACTORS OF EARLY CHILDHOOD

Many significant changes are required of families as children enter the family system. Parents adjust the marital dyad to make space for new family members, the parenting role is gradually learned, and relationships with extended family members are realigned in order to include the parental and grandparental roles (Carter & McGoldrick, 1980). While these family changes are negotiated, the married couple must also take care to attend to their relationship, and the solo parent must develop and maintain adult relationships. Life becomes more complex as a newly created two generation system negotiates the paradigmatic shifts in thinking and behaving that accompany the integration of new members into the system. Nevertheless, families who enjoy a history of successful problem-solving and whose economic resources are adequate will move through the transition with a fair amount of ease. The complexity of the transition, however, may become overwhelming to families lacking in problem-solving skills, living in poverty, or struggling to maintain a minimally adequate standard of living.

The New Family Member

As parents make space for children, their foreknowledge of developmental expectations is helpful but seldom fully prepares them for the advent of the new family member. Several family specialists have used the term "crisis" to describe the birth or adoption of the first child (LeMasters, 1957; Burr, 1972; Dyer, 1963). Family disruption, chronic fatigue, and the temperament of the infant are some of the factors that affect parents as they accommodate to their new family member. As the child matures and additional children join the family, new challenges confront parents as they attempt to deal with the rapidly evolving developmental milestones associated with the early childhood years. In addition, couples with young children generally report lower marital satisfaction than do couples in later stages of the family life cycle (Rollins & Feldman, 1970). These developmental issues, along with the countless joys and pleasures associated with the early childhood years, are common in families whose children are "normal." The disruption of developmental delay or disability adds significantly to the problems with which families must deal during these early years.

When a child is born with a developmental disability or when a problem is identified during the early years, family members must deal with the "loss of the dream" (Moses, 1985). Their dream of the perfect child, once envisioned, is destroyed and the family must begin the slow process of getting to know this "new" child. Speech-language pathologists working with families during this time will encounter parents at various stages in the loss process who are also dealing with other issues of development associated with this child, as well as parenting their other children. Understanding the context or milieu in which early intervention services are provided gives the clinician a deeper understanding and comprehension of the possible effects of his words, non verbal behaviors, and attitude on the child and family.

One situation, encountered to some extent by nearly all families confronted with early childhood delay and disability, is the plethora of differing professional opinions that parents must sort through in order to make wise decisions regarding treatment. Few families have had any preparation for dealing with this complex array of advice, often presented with a certainty that is simultaneously overwhelming and confusing. The fortunate parents who feel certain about what is best for their child, or who encounter a professional that is supportive of their efforts to maintain their appropriate role as decision-makers, will be empowered and strengthened as they deal with the challenges and joys of parenting a young child. This sense of competence will be conveyed to the child who will, in turn, benefit from the stability offered by the self-confident parents.

Finally, as the family accommodates to its new member, the nagging uncertainty of the eventual outcome of the effects of the delay or disability may be an added stressor. As the child matures his/her potential becomes clearer, but during the early years uncertainty often prevails. Some families are unable to get an exact diagnosis of the problem or may be given several different diagnoses. Even when the diagnosis is clear, the prognosis is often less certain. Family-Based Treatment gives the family permission to struggle with the clinician in a partnership of honesty, hope, setbacks, and successes as, together, they work to create positive changes and adaptations so that the child's potential during the early years of development is realized.

New Couple and Parenting Roles

When a child is born into a family, the married couple has to change their way of relating to one another. If the parent is a solo parent, it becomes necessary to adapt to an individually oriented adult lifestyle while learning to parent the child alone unless grandparents, siblings, or friends are available for help and support. All through the family life cycle, the importance of maintaining satisfying and enriching adult relationships is vital to the well-being of parents who, in turn, are strengthened to provide the nurturing and care that is vital to the well-being of their children. This task can be a particularly arduous one for families having a young child with special needs.

The task of maintaining the couple relationship is especially challenging when one parent is responsible for taking the child to appointments with professionals and then attempts to follow the prescribed directives of each of these professionals while translating that information to the spouse or other family members. In many two-parent families the mother accepts this role while the father focuses his energy on work and career demands. Some mothers are forced to temporarily give up or cut back on their career plans as caregiving responsibilities become a priority. Other mothers must figure out how to meet job responsibilities while also attending to the frequent professional appointments engendered by their children's special needs. The speech-language pathologist can make a significant contribution to the well-being of families in the early childhood years by arranging appointments at times that are convenient to *both* parents. Fathers are willing participants when it is clear that their involvement is useful and wanted. Only once in eighteen years have we had a father in a two-parent family turn down our invitation to participate in treatment. Our efforts to enlist fathers on the treatment team have paid off in benefits to their children, enrichment of our treatment planning, and cohesiveness of the family as the couple engages in mutual decision-making relative to their child. In fact, when entire families participate, there is evidence that they begin to think of speech-language services as a family activity. One family member expressed it this way: "Right now, it is just something we do; our family goes to speech therapy. All the kids go, but she (child with a disability) is not different." Another said, ". . . basically, it has been fun to have it be something the whole family does instead of just something that one of the kids has an appointment to do. More an activity that feels like the family being together." And, finally, "I think it is important for us to be there and work more with us and the issues that go on behind the scenes, so to speak, of the speech problem . . . and I think it kind of treats us as a family, and it is a family deal. Dawn is the main thing, but it affects our family" (Fehsenfeld, et al., 1996).

If the child lives in a solo-parent family and if the custodial parent agrees, we always ask the child's non-custodial parent to join the treatment team. Parents, of course, may not be married to one another, but they never divorce their children and usually want to remain active in the child's life. We also like to include grandparents, aunts, uncles, live-in friends, and other supportive individuals who are available to assist the solo parent and/or who may have direct influence on the treatment of the communicative disorder. These individuals can, at the parents' request, act as co-parents with the busy parent of a preschooler and offer valuable support as the speech-language disorder is treated.

Sometimes professionals become overzealous in their desire to promote change and expect parents to provide almost constant reinforcement and stimulation to their children. In our experience, it is much more useful to be sensitive to potential parental exhaustion and suggest that it might be best for the child if the parents took a night out or arranged for time together and focused on their own adult interests. This time "away" can help parents refuel and develop renewed energy for the challenges presented by a child with special needs.

Finally, children will benefit when clinicians support parents in their appropriate role and carefully guard parents' rights to make decisions about their children. These decisions will not always be the same as those the professional would like parents to make, but unless the clinician plans to be responsible for the child until the child reaches maturity or is no longer in need of services, that right is the parents' alone. We must take great care to avoid usurping the parental role. Instead, we should support and enhance the interactive resources that parents bring to treatment. This concept has been expressed as empowerment (Dunst, Trivette, et al. (1988), and the word has become familiar to all who provide early intervention services. Unfortunately, we have heard some clinicians express dismay when the term is used. We are never quite sure whether their negative reaction is to the word itself or to the concept that the word represents. Although some may tire of hearing the word, the concept represents, for us, the cornerstone of early intervention and the manner in which all services should be provided.

The Extended Family

When a first child is born, parents are also "born." In some cases, grandparents are created for the first time. Even if the couple has had few expressed differences prior to the birth of the child, differences are very likely to emerge at this point. Each parent was parented by different people, and grandparental opinions often become a significant part of the family system at this point. When parents are confident, supportive of one another, able to deal with differences, and can enlist the grandparents as *consultants* to the parenting process, the transition will be fairly smooth. Extended family conflict can erupt, however, if grandparents become uninvited experts who disqualify the fledgling parents as they are learning their new role. Such conflict, if not resolved after the birth of the first child, continues both overtly and covertly with the birth of subsequent children. Again, the introduction of new grandparents, great grandparents, aunts, and uncles into a family can be a stressful process when the child shows no unusual problems. When developmental delay or disability is evident, the differences between the parents themselves and between parents, grandparents, and other significant family members may become more apparent.

Extended family members are important additions to the treatment team when their presence is desired by the parent or parents. If the parent is a solo parent, grandparents and great-grandparents often have frequent contact with the child and are able to offer significant assistance as strategies for change are identified. All decisions, however, must be finally approved by the parent so that her role as the primary caregiver of her child is strengthened. Ordinarily, we begin treatment with the child and parent alone unless they are living in the grandparental home. When the grandparents have knowledge, resources, and influence that can be accessed for speech-language change, it is a good idea to enlist their participation in the decision-making process, but to remember to respect the parent's role and be sensitive to the extent to which she wants to be in charge. Actions as simple as beginning an interview by learning the parent's perspective first or making a positive comment about the parent to the grandparents at an appropriate time, give evidence to the clinician's assumption that the parent is in charge. These strategic actions must, however, be done in a manner that is respectful of everyone present; they will be most successful when that is the clinician's genuine intention.

When working with two-parent families, after several sessions and when we feel joined with the parents, we frequently ask about the reactions of grandparents if the topic has not already been discussed. If intergenerational differences appear to be focused on reactions and responses to the child's speech-language situation, we work with the parents to plan a three-generational meeting in which the goals of treatment are described and the grandparents' resources are identified. The act of convening this large group of people, all of whom love and care for the child in question, usually eases the intergenerational conflict and produces new ideas for change.

In most cases, however, the three or four generations of each family are already joined in their concern for the well-being of the child with a communicative disorder even before the speech-language pathologist enlists their support. When this reciprocal love and concern is accessed and recognized, possibilities for change are expanded, and the child benefits greatly.

EARLY INTERVENTION CASE STUDIES

The three case studies presented below illustrate some of the principles of systemic, family-centered, solution-focused early intevention services using the Family-Based Treatment process model. All three case studies illustrate the concepts of identifying and building on family resources and developing isomorphic assignments. Scaling communicative behavior, as described in Chapter 4, is illustrated in the first case study. Responding to the grief process and enabling a parent are particularly prominent features of the second example. The clinician's use of self and the influence of stressors in the life of the family with young children are illustrated in the third case study.

Case Study 1: Family Participation in Assessment and Using Scaling to Set Goals

Jonah was 24 months old, and his parents were concerned because he was using only a few words. He was referred for an evaluation by the initial service coordinator in our county who is responsible for obtaining assessments and securing services for those infants and toddlers found to be eligible.

Jonah was accompanied to the speech-language assessment by his mother, father, and 9-year-old sister, Naomi. His parents were concerned that he wasn't using many words and that when he did use words he said only a fragment of the word rather than the entire word. They said Jonah responded best to his sister and that she often was successful in encouraging him to imitate words. Jonah's communication consisted largely of pointing and gesturing or saying part of a word and gesturing. Activities his parents had done to help him included naming objects to which he was attending; repeating words Jonah said; and playing with a toy microphone, a game that Jonah's sister invented. Jonah vocalized readily when holding the microphone and playing a talking game with his sister.

As a way of introducing the child to us, Jonah's mother showed Jonah pictures in a book. Naomi stood close by and looked on. Naomi frequently said the name of the picture when Johah didn't and asked Jonah to say it; he often did, although many consonants were omitted and his consonantal repertoire seemed limited. When he said words, Jonah's mother repeated them. We commented on Jonah's mother's naming pictures at which he was looking, following his lead as she turned the pages, allowing Naomi to be part of the activity, repeating words Jonah said, and helping Jonah continue to enjoy the activity without becoming frustrated by Naomi's request for Jonah to name pictures. We briefly discussed these characteristics as well as Jonah's production of words, the sounds we heard, and his willingness to imitate Naomi. Many family resources, or mobilization points, were becoming evident. At this point, we asked Jonah's mother to show him pictures on the *Structured Photographic Articulation Test (SPAT-D)* (Kresheck and Werner, 1989). We all listened, attending particularly to sounds we heard Jonah use. A profile of Jonah's sound repertoire and usage, as well as his use of expressive language, began to develop. Both Jonah's father and sister sat closely and were attentively involved, as were we, as Jonah named the pictures and talked about them. We commented frequently on what we heard as Jonah's articulatory repertoire was being discovered so that Jonah's father and mother could learn about Jonah's speech and language from our perspective. We encouraged Jonah and Naomi to play as we described the inventory we would use next. A copy of the *Rossetti Infant-Toddler Language Scale* (Rossetti, 1990) was given to each parent. We began at the 12-15 month level and discussed the items in the Language Expression portion of the inventory. From time to time, Jonah entered our conversation, and we used some of these times to "try out" an item. Both the clinician and Jonah's parents participated in asking Jonah to do this. His father, for example, asked Jonah to imitate him as he made the sounds of a lion, a dog, and a cat. The family took a copy of the Scale home to think about some more, and we agreed to meet again the following week. We also sent home a copy of *The MacArthur Communicative Development Inventory: Words and Gestures* (Fenson, et al.,1993) for the parents to begin completing.

Prior to the family's leaving, we encouraged them to continue imitating words Jonah said, to show him that they were happy when he says words, and to pay attention to consonant sounds they heard Jonah using, particularly those that we hadn't heard during the session. The latter, of course, was a continuation of what we had discussed as Jonah named pictures on the articulation test. Finally, the clinician encouraged them to continue with the microphone game and for Naomi, along with her parents, to imitate words and sounds Jonah said on his turn with the microphone. We continued to learn about Jonah's speech-language level at the next session, while beginning treatment. We learned enough by the end of the second session to write a report about Jonah's expressive language to qualify him for early intervention services. Additional information was gathered at each subsequent session.

In order to set short and long term goals for Jonah, we engaged the family in scaling Jonah's communication at the second session. The clinician began as follows:

> Clinician: Here's a different way to think about Jonah's speech and language. We could put his communication on a one to ten-point scale with 1 being where he was when you called for the appointment and 10 being what his speech and language will be like when you think he's on track and won't need services anymore. So . . . let's think about what he was like when we first talked on the telephone. We'll call that a 1.

Jonah's parents both participated in sharing information. Since the first telephone contact had not occurred long before (e.g., about two weeks), their descriptions were not significantly different from what we had seen at session one. Both parents were, however, able to talk about Jonah's speech-language in a knowledgeable manner after having participated in our initial assessment. After Jonah's parents described Jonah's communicative ability at the time of our initial telephone conversation, the clinician asked them to describe their idea of a 10. Notice that the act of describing Jonah's speech-language reinforces the information they participated in gathering at the first session and contributes to making them good observers of their son's speech-language development.

> Clinician: OK, we've said that the behavior you just described defines a 1 on the scale of 1 to 10. Jonah was . . . (summarizes what the parents said) . . . Now, let's think about what Jonah will be like when you'll feel satisfied with his speech and language. At that point, you may decide that he doesn't need services any longer. We'll rate that behavior at 10.

The act of describing what Jonah will be like when his parents are satisfied with his speech, presupposes that such a time will come. In Jonah's case, we can be reasonably certain that he will fall within normal limits at that time, even though his parents may not require perfection. Other parents whose children are more severely delayed have been remarkably developmentally appropriate when describing a 10 for their child.

Jonah's parents described a time when Jonah would be speaking so that everyone could understand what he was saying, when he would be using sentences like other children his age, and when he could talk with his grandparents on the telephone, and they wouldn't ask him to repeat because they could understand him. The clinician accepted the parents' descriptions non judgmentally and used clarification and reflection to assure that she understood what they meant.

> Clinician: You'll be satisfied with Jonah's speech and language when . . . (summarizes what the parents have described) . . .We'll call that a 10. We have descriptions of 1, when you first called for an appointment and 10, when you'll be satisfied with Jonah's speech. Let's use your description of Jonah's speech when you would be satisfied as our long-term goal.

The next step is for the family to establish a number between 1 and 10 that represents Jonah's speech-language today. They have participated in the the assessment (and will continue to participate as additional information about Jonah's speech-language emerges and is sought during treatment). The clinician initiates a brief discussion about Jonah's present level:

> Clinician: Let's talk about what Jonah's speech and language is like right now. We've found that . . . (describes findings; parents participate by adding information) . . . Where, on that 1 to 10 scale, would you place Jonah right now?

Jonah's parents discussed this briefly. His mother rated his communication at a 3 and his father rated it at 4. There is no right or wrong answer! The clinician accepted both ratings and moved to the next step:

> Clinician: OK, (to the mother) for you, Jonah's speech and language right now is at a 3, and (to the father) for you, Jonah is communicating at a 4. Now, what would he be doing (to mother) if he were at 3 1/2 or 4 or (to father) 4 1/2 or 5? In other words, what would he have to do to move up one-half point, or even one point on your scales?

> Father: I think if he'd start using those back sounds you talked about, you know, "k" and "g" that he'd move up one-half point.

> Mother: Well, I don't know; I think I'd rather see him use more words and start putting words together to make sentences. I think if he said words more readily, for example, when we're looking at books, I'd move him up one-half point or even one point if he named a lot of things.

Clinician: We can work in both of these areas. These will be our short-term goals: Jonah will use the "k" and "g" sounds in, how many words shall we say?

Father: Well, I think if we could get him to use each of them in five to ten words, he'd be on the way.

Clinician: OK, let's say that one of our goals is for Jonah to use the "k" in five words and the "g" sound in five words. What about using more words? How will we know if he's using more words?

Mother: I look at those books so often, I pretty much know the pictures he names. Maybe I could tell you any new words he uses.

Clinician: Good, you'll keep track of new words Jonah uses, maybe write them down, and when he uses what shall we say, ten, you'll raise his level one-half point.

Mother: Well, I was thinking fifteen, but maybe I'll go with ten.

The short-term goals are now set. The next task is for the clinican to search for exceptions and determine if the new behavior *ever* occurs and, if so, under what circumstances. Following this, and building upon the exceptions, if possible, the clinician and family will determine the procedures they'll use to facilitate and elicit the new behaviors. This, of course, makes up the assignment.

Clinician: Let's talk about Jonah using the "k" and "g" sounds. Has there ever been a time when he's used one of these? Are there any times when he comes close to using one?

Father: I've heard him use "k" once, about three or four weeks ago. He said 'key' as I was opening the front door, and I said something like, 'I can't find my key.' I did eventually find it, but I'm pretty sure he said the word.

Clinician: Let's see if you can get him to say it right now. OK?

Father: Sure. (father calls Jonah over, gets his attention, and exaggerates the "k" as he says 'key' and asks Jonah to say it. After four trials, Jonah still does not use it in the word 'key.'

Clinician: How about, this week you not ask Jonah to say any words, but rather, as you interact with him, exaggerate the way you say the "k" just as you did when you asked Jonah to say it. This will call it to his attention . . . it will highlight it for him kind of like we do when we use a highlighter on printed words.

Father: OK, I can do that. I'll find excuses to use k-words and exaggerate them. But, shouldn't I try to get him to say it too?

Clinician: Since he can't do it, I think it would be better for you to call the sound to his attention by exaggerating it. If he says it, however, let him know you're really happy . . . really praise him. Even if he doesn't say it, your highlighting it for him may make it easier for us to elicit next week during our session. Now (to mother), he already does use some words and names some of the pictures as you look at books with him. What you did here (the clinician has the benefit of having watched the mother during the initial assessment) was follow his lead and talk about pictures he's interested in. You did it in a really calm way and Naomi helped by asking Jonah to say words. Here are two ideas: Sometimes, when you're looking at the book and naming the pictures, Naomi could ask him to say one of the words. When he does (to mother), you praise Jonah; let him know you're really happy, and say the word two or three more times. Encourage him to watch your face when you do that. Naomi, you can clap and let him know you're happy too, and (back to mother) repeat the word several times as you encourage Jonah to look at you. He may even say it again. If he does, let him know you're happy and repeat it again. At other times, name the pictures as you do, and point to some of them as you name them. Once in a while, when you come to the picture of a word you know he says, say something like, "Here's a . . ." and pause as you point, giving Jonah an opportunity to say the word. When he's accustomed to the technique, begin pausing occasionally on some of the words you are sure he knows, but hasn't said. If you pause and Jonah doesn't say the word, you go ahead and say it. If he does say it, let him know you're happy and repeat it like we already talked about. How does that sound?

Mother: Good.

Clinician: Let's try it for a minute or two and see how it looks.

Both long and short-term goals have been set, the family is "on board," and an isomorphic, systemic, polyocular assignment for each family member has been developed. The clinician will experiment very briefly with the assignment given to the mother and Naomi to observe what happens when they enact the suggestion. This will give the clinician an opportunity to "fine tune" the assignment if it doesn't work out as planned and Jonah's mother and sister an opportunity to practice in a situation where friendly feedback may be given.

In this case study, the clinician has provided opportunities for family members to show their abilities and resources and develop new ones to meet the needs of their child. The family members all showed their abilities as they participated in the assessment. The mobilization points identified during the assessment were utilized in the assignment developed after the family set Jonah's long and short-term goals. We are continuing to learn about the effectiveness of having family members scale speech-language. Our belief is that it has significant possiblilities for engaging family members in the goal setting process.

Case Study #2: Responding to the Grieving Process

Parents, siblings, grandparents, and other relatives of a child born with a cleft lip and/or palate or any craniofacial anomaly are confronted with the physical evidence of the problem on the day of birth. The joyful preparation, excitement, tension, physical pain, and tremendous relief associated with childbirth are suddenly obliterated by shock, grief, fear, and an overwhelming sorrow. Professionals and family members wanting to console the grieving parents often make the mistake of downplaying the tragedy assuring them that surgery will correct nature's error and that things are not really so bad. Even worse, these people may tiptoe around the issue speaking in hushed tones as they try to protect the exhausted mother from the reality of the situation by avoiding discussion of the event. Others may tell the parents how they "should" respond, thus further negating the right of the parents to express their grief in their own manner. One mother of a child born with a cleft palate told us that a hospital professional had admonished her that she was not grieving properly because no one had seen her cry since the birth of her daughter. This statement further compounded her grief and left her with feelings of hurt and anger toward the insensitive professional.

More fortunate families are offered the opportunity to interact with professionals who quietly attend to their needs as the numbness subsides; who allow them to express their grief, anger, and pain; and who answer all questions honestly and simply as they arise. From the beginning of their child's life, these families are encouraged to be active participants as decisions are made. The well-being of the child is related to the well-being of the parents, and specialists in cleft palate emphasize the importance of the professional's willingness to work with family members as treatment plans are developed for the young child with a cleft lip and/or palate (Goetz, 1982; Hahn, 1979; Schwartz, 1982). These families are beginning the process of empowerment that will enable them to trust their own abilities and feelings as they face the difficult days ahead.

Michael's mother describes her reaction to the array of services and decisions that confronted her during her first months and early years with her son:

When my child was born, I had no knowledge of the extensive treatment that was involved in his medical care. There were surgeries, orthodontics, speech therapy, ear problems and emotional development to consider. I had to rely mainly on each specialist to provide me with the necessary information needed for his growth. What I encountered was a mixture of 'professional egotism' from some of the specialists and a genuine concern for Michael's well-being from others.

Michael's surgeon insisted that he be seen by a clinic that could provide a "Team Approach". After attending the first clinic, I was told that an evaluation would be sent to me of each professional's opinion. When I read the report, I didn't understand it. It was written by professionals for professionals. When I tried to have the report explained to me, some of the specialists told me to just keep bringing him for the evaluations, and they would take care of it. They knew how to treat a cleft palate child. They had worked with 6000 before. The problem was that I didn't know how or what they were treating him for. Was it possible for me to enhance areas of his development? Would I do something to retard his development? I had no way of knowing. I sought second and sometimes third opinions to become more knowledgeable of options available to my child.

When Michael was about to begin speech therapy I heard of a clinic that incorporated the family in the treatment. It was explained to me that therapy would be enhanced if the family members understood objectives and could help the child in his speech development. The results have been astounding. We, the professionals, the parent, and the child, as a team, have been able to accomplish goals necessary for Michael's well-being.

Though the results of his speech have been positive, not all other aspects are. I still find it a struggle to be incorporated in other areas of his care. There are choices, and as a parent I want to make competent decisions concerning my son's treatment. It is important to remember that each child is an individual and not just another case to be handled. The parent is as necessary as each specialist in overall treatment. Without the two working together, the child ultimately suffers, and the professional's knowledge has been of no use. (Seibel, 1987a, p.1-2)

Michael's mother, Nancy, contacted the clinician when Michael was 20 months old. She wanted services for Michael, and a state agency that funds children's speech-language services when they are secondary to health or physical problems, agreed to pay for these services. Nancy was a veteran visitor to specialists but was tentatively enthusiastic about the possibility of being more involved in the decision-making process. Her considerable energy and strong desire to remain in charge of decisions relating to her son were viewed by the clinician as assets. She and Michael's father had divorced a year earlier. Since that time Michael had almost no contact with his father, and apparently no child support was forthcoming. Our suggestion that father be included in the sessions was not supported by Nancy, and her wishes were respected since she was the custodial parent. Mother and son were living with the maternal grandparents and also in close proximity to the maternal great-grandmother. This excellent support system benefited Michael since he was surrounded by many loving adults. Both grandmothers, as well as Nancy's brother, participated in sessions when Nancy felt that this was appropriate.

Michael, a blond, shy toddler was born with a complete bilateral cleft lip and palate. The cleft lip and palate had been surgically repaired although scarring in the the area of the lip was clearly evident. Michael, clearly wary of another "Doctor," observed most of the first session from a safe corner of the room, responding with tears when interaction with the clinician was requested. Michael's normal fears were respected, and most of the first session focused on data gathering as Nancy described the speech and language characteristics that she had noticed, as well as her hopes for her son's development. Toward the end of the session, Michael approached his mother, and she was able to elicit from him some of the speech responses necessary for a beginning assessment of his situation.

As the beginning phase of treatment evolved, Michael's shyness disappeared and a bright, assertive toddler emerged. The primary goal was for Michael to develop an oral air stream for speech and to make full use of his velopharyngeal mechanism. If surgery had given him an adequate mechanism, he would learn to use it. If the mechanism were inadequate, that would become increasingly apparent. Secondary goals were to facilitate further language development and to increase mobility of his upper lip. Nancy was actively involved in a number of activities designed to meet these goals. Helping Michael increase the variety of consonant sounds by letting him watch her face and touch her lips while she blew, said babababa, papapapa, etc. and made other noises are examples of beginning procedures. Weekly sessions were held and, at each session, goals and procedures were altered and changed to fit Nancy and Michael's interactive style and to elicit speech-language change. Michael's language development improved significantly. Changes in speech continued to be characterized by hypernasality and nasal air emission, but Michael's considerable effort and Nancy's continuing work with him at home increased the variety of places of articulation that Michael used.

As Michael matured and became more verbal and Nancy became very expert in her ability to reinforce his appropriate speech utterances, we began to space sessions farther apart since her use of reinforcement in the natural context was providing the stimulation that he needed. The clinician believed that a surgical re-evaluation was necessary because all best efforts did not seem to bring the mechanism to its desired functioning for speech purposes. A meeting with the surgeon and Nancy was held, and the decision was made to delay work on the velopharyngeal mechanism until cosmetic revision of Michael's lip was completed. The cosmetic surgery was subsequently performed necessitating a vacation from speech-language treatment and altering the amount of effort that young Michael could muster for articulatory practice.

Following the "vacation," Family-Based Treatment resumed, and Michael's articulatory competence continued to improve. This competence, however, was not at a level expected, and surgery was scheduled to construct and place a pharyngeal flap. Meanwhile, an orthodontic evaluation was conducted, and plans were made to prevent collapse of the alveolar ridge segments. Throughout all of these changes, speech-language treatment had to be suspended as medical and dental treatment were implemented. Nancy, however, now very knowledgeable about speech change, continued to help Michael when it was clear to her that he was physically able to be involved in attention to speech. Michael had evolved into a bright, intelligent, perceptive three-year-old who was comfortable with himself in spite of the regime of treatments he endured.

As these changes occurred, Michael also was enrolled in preschool, and Nancy returned to work, at first part-time and then on a full-time basis. She and Michael moved to an apartment of their own while grandmother and great-grandmother continued to assist with child care when Nancy's work schedule required such assistance. Michael began developing friendships, and Nancy was finally able to schedule some personal recreation time into her life. A "normal" life style began to emerge. Meanwhile, speech-language services were maintained through monthly visits. During these sessions Nancy would report and demonstrate the interactive speech-language techniques that she was using, and the clinician would then suggest new procedures as needed.

When Michael entered kindergarten, Nancy decided that he should continue speech-language treatment at school, and contact was made with the speech-language clinician to assure a smooth transition and to encourage the inclusion of Michael's mother in the treatment process at school. Nancy's confident, competent parenting, as well as her thorough knowledge of Michael's speech-language needs and velopharyngeal capabilities, empowered her to continue to make the necessary decisions associated with her maturing son. Again, the reader is privileged to share Nancy's experience as she describes her personal responses to these early years with Michael.

As an expectant parent, I was filled with feelings of excitement, anticipation and joy. I was going to be a mother. Will it be a boy or girl? What will we name it? Who will it look like? What a happy time this was and what a tremendous disappointment when I found out he was born less that perfect.

When the doctor told me that my baby had been born with a bilateral cleft lip and palate, I felt absolutely devastated to see him so severely deformed. I couldn't believe that this had happened to me. Why was God punishing me? I had always heard that there was an immediate bond between a mother and her child. This simply wasn't the case for me; I felt no love for this baby; I felt nothing.

After I returned to my room, people would call me and tell me to thank God it wasn't a heart defect or some other problem. However, that was no consolation to me. You can't see a heart defect, but you could see his facial disfigurement. No one ever congratulated me on his birth. When my husband saw him, he said, 'Oh, it's no big deal.' My God what was he saying? Was I the only one feeling devastated, shocked and scared? How could I possibly cope?

The surgeon came in and told me Michael would never look "normal," never like you and me, but a repair would be done. Oh, my God, this won't go away will it? What am I going to do? He told me that the baby must weigh ten pounds before the closure could be done. 'Go home and enjoy your son.' How could I possibly do that? How could I possibly enjoy this baby? How could I possibly love this child? Throughout my hospital stay my husband only came up once.

When I brought Michael home, I wasn't sure I could care for him; I wasn't sure I wanted to. As I went through the motions, I began to notice what pretty blue eyes he had, his beautiful strawberry blonde hair, and then I saw him smile. Michael was real; he was alive, and I was hurting deeply.

At two months, Michael was ready for his first surgery, and so was I. After waiting for three hours, the surgeon came out very excited with the results. He quickly brought me to the recovery room to show me. What I saw was my baby with a lip. He was crying and had several stitches. They brought him to his room and asked me to hold him. I was scared. I didn't know how to care for him. The nurses helped me, and I did fine. My husband never came to see him. When the swelling went down and sutures removed, I had his first picture taken.

In the next few months, I began to really enjoy Michael. He started to crawl, then walk and eventually he said 'Mama'. I never thought I could be so excited. However, the excitement was mixed with fear. My husband and I divorced. Would I be able to care for Michael and myself financially and emotionally? I knew I would do my best.

Michael had his fourth surgery at two and one-half years years of age. The first night was always the hardest, but when Michael woke up and was crying, 'No more, Mommy, no more. I promise I will be a good boy,' I hated myself for putting him through an elective cosmetic surgery. Why did I still care what he looked like? I loved him or thought I did. I looked out the window of the hospital and wanted to jump. I can't do it anymore. I couldn't bear to know that he thought I was punishing him. I honestly did love him. I sought professional help for my emotional well-being and for his.

In the past five years, I have learned to deal with the added pressures of a special child. I have found that I love Michael for who he is and not just for what he looks like, and in turn he loves me for those same reasons. It has not been easy, and I am sure I will continue to have difficult times, but now I know that God gave me a son that is absolutely everything that I could have asked for and more. I realize God gave me the perfect child, and I am capable of a love that I never knew existed. (Seibel, 1987b)

Nancy's eloquent sharing of her personal journey, not yet completed, reminds each of us of our professional responsibility to attend to the feelings, needs, and parenting potential of the mothers of our preschool clients.

Case Study # 3: Using the "Self of the Clinician" to Guide Treatment

We view Family-Based Treatment as a refinement of traditional treatment of early stuttering since the home environment and family interactions have received attention for many years (Van Riper, 1954). Often, mothers meet with the speech-language pathologist, and fathers and siblings are not involved in treatment. Further, family interactions may be described as they are experienced by the mother, but since the rest of the family is not present, interactions are seldom observed, and the perspectives of other family members are not heard. Family-Based Treatment expands the treatment possibilities since the speech-language pathologist has the benefit of a polyocular view, has access to family resources, directly observes family interactions, and tracks other interactive events.

As the speech-language pathologist joins the family system and participates in the family's interactions, the clinician may sense and be affected by the emotions or feelings of family members. The same pressures, playfulness, anxiety, defensiveness, elation, depression, etc. felt by family members are often felt by the clinician. When the clinician attends to these feelings, she can use her reactions as information to help her make decisions about her role in treatment. This process is called "use of self" (see Chapter 8). It is especially useful in cases of early stuttering because it gives the clinician additional, although very subjective, information about what the child may be experiencing. When there is tension between parents, pressure on a child to "be correct" or to react in particular pre-set structured ways, or competition between family members, etc. the child is likely to sense this and respond to it. Just as it is not uncommon for the clinician to feel this to the point that his own participation in interactions are tempered in order to be "appropriate," the child is likely doing the same thing but at a more rudimentary level. The ways in which these feelings and attitudes are manifested in family interactions may be the critical point. For example, when the content of parent-child play is limited to opportunities to educate the child, and the interactions of play consist primarily of asking the child questions or telling him facts, the child who is experiencing early stuttering may feel pressure just as the clinician who attempts to play with the child "in the correct way" will feel pressure. The climate of interaction in such a case may be a variable which could be changed and manipulated in an effort to influence fluency.

We also suggest that the *normal* parental conflict experienced by parents during the early years may affect speech fluency in the child who is predisposed to early stuttering. This conflict can affect the parents' ability to provide consistent structure for the child. The child, in turn, may become confused and agitated thus, creating a situation that is not conducive to effective communication. Access to such interactions and accommodation of parental differences may influence fluency modification efforts.

Kyle was 31 months, nearly three years old, when he was identified through the early intervention screening program. He passed all aspects of the screening areas except speech-language and was referred for an assessment. Kyle's family consisted of his mother; his father, who had himself received treatment for stuttering and articulation as a child; and his seven-year-old brother. The family was convened shortly after we received the referral; all family members attended the first session and understood that the purpose was to learn more about Kyle's fluency and determine his eligibility for early intervention services.

It was apparent at the outset that conversation in Kyle's family was frequent and fast-paced. Kyle's mother was the family spokesperson and talked a lot. During the first session the only pressure felt by the clinician was that he had to work very hard to participate as a speaker rather than strictly a listener. Kyle's brother talked a lot, too. He and Kyle played together during a good part of the first session. Kyle showed little indication of monitoring our conversation, but his brother was obviously doing so and sometimes corrected his parents about the details of family events they described. Kyle's father spoke infrequently. Both he and Kyle often had their conversational turns usurped or cut short by someone interrupting them. Still, the clinician felt comfortable interacting with the family, and the parents seemed accepting of both boys. No particular stress or tension was apparent even though conversational "space" was limited due to the mother's ability to talk in an animated and fast-paced manner.

Consistent with the high value placed on conversation, the family did not own a television set. They valued education and self development highly; both parents were professors. Both showed acceptance of Kyle and talked about his assets which included being a relaxed and comfortable child. Family members enjoyed his company. Both parents were concerned about Kyle's fluency, but both also felt that he would likely become more fluent since that had been the father's experience. Both parents likened Kyle to his father and Kyle's brother to his mother.

Family resources evident at the first session included the fact that the family enjoyed playing games together, that both boys liked to read or be read to and that this occurred nearly every evening. Also, Kyle was "easy going" and seldom became upset, Kyle's brother liked to play with him and was generally helpful by nature, and the parents self-reported that mother talked a lot. They agreed that they both talked fast even though they thought that perhaps they should try to speak more slowly.

Kyle had repetitions of sounds and syllables on five to eight percent of his words. Tension in muscles of his neck accompanied some of his disfluencies.

During the first session, the clinician played a game of checkers with Kyle and spoke very little. All of the clinician's talking was at a reduced though natural rate. He paid particular attention to allowing pause time after Kyle had spoken. Both parents and Kyle's brother watched the game. At one time or another, all gave Kyle advice; the clinician did not respond to this. The room was noticeably quiet during the game, particularly in contrast to the previous thirty minutes when the parents were being interviewed. After the game the adults discussed what had occurred, and both parents expressed surprise that an adult could play with a child and keep the child's interest without talking most of the time. This idea formed the basis for the first assignment which was isomorphic to the parents' expression that they should probably slow the rate of their own speech. It was polyocular in that they had experienced a new way of interacting with a child which included a slow, conversational rate with reduced verbal output and an absence of questions. The assignment was systemic in that a slower rate of speech was to be incorporated into natural interactions with Kyle. The specific assignment was to do the following:

> For about fifteen minutes each day, try to speak slowly when interacting with Kyle. As you suggested, this could be done when you are looking at books with him. Modify the length of time up or down to fit your schedule and notice:
>
> 1. Is this possible to do?
>
> 2. What is the effect on Kyle's speech? (eg., Did he slow his rate, too? Were disfluencies evident? Did he talk more? Less? etc.)

Subsequent sessions consisted of an elaboration of this theme of rate of speech and pause-time, use of questions by the parents, and attention to turn-taking interactions. Techniques for maintaining Kyle's feeling of self-worth in relation to his brother were discussed and other variables possibly related to periods of disfluency were examined. Kyle's parents were rewarded for their insights into Kyle's disfluency and for their ability to notice potential fluency disrupters. Isomorphic, polyocular, and systemic assignments were carried out by the family.

Predictably, Kyle's fluency varied over the ten-month period. One week when Kyle had been ill and was still weak, his disfluencies were especially severe. At the same time, his family noticed that they did have influence over other situations that seemed related to disfluency. They noticed that when they stopped interrupting Kyle and gave him plenty of time to complete his conversational turn, when they rewarded his efforts to be appropriately in charge or in control of his life, and when they reduced the number of questions they asked him, his fluency improved. Other effective techniques included reducing their own amount of talking and their requests for Kyle to talk during periods of disfluency, ignoring some of Kyle's articulation errors rather than attempting to correct them, and preparing Kyle for anticipated changes in routine.

Kyle and his family were seen each week during the summer for six one-hour sessions. We continued to work with them for an additional ten sessions after school began in the fall. These ten sessions were spread over an eight month period. In all, the family was seen by us for seventeen one-hour sessions over a period of eleven months. Kyle also received treatment at school from the speech-language pathologist when school resumed in the fall. While our primary focus of concern, by mutual agreement, was fluency, at school the clinician's focus of concern was articulation and speech intelligibility. This was a general guideline, however, and we each monitored both communicative behaviors and could not help but overlap occasionally in our efforts. Treatment with us was terminated at the seventeenth session by mutual agreement. Kyle's parents had heard no stuttering for over a month and felt that they were capable of controlling the stuttering through adjusting the environment if the disfluencies returned. The speech-language pathologist at Kyle's school agreed and continued to work with Kyle on articulation. This provided an opportunity for another person to monitor Kyle's fluency. Three years post-treatment, Kyle was a fluent and intelligible speaker and a slightly above-average student. His parents enjoyed the satisfaction of having helped their own child, and it seemed that their feelings of competence would likely generalize to other inevitable and normal problem situations that would arise before Kyle reached adulthood.

SUMMARY

Families with young children must accommodate to the rapidly changing physical, social, and emotional needs of their children. The well-being of the child is powerfully influenced by the well-being of his/her parents. Therefore, adults must assure that their own needs are met. When a child is born with special needs, these developmental tasks are complicated by the extra attention that the child must receive and the decisions that must be made relative to professional intervention.

Involving the family in treatment ensures their rightful place in the decision-making process and enhances the clinician's opportunities to create assignments that will benefit the child. The Family-Based Treatment model can be used to guide early interventionists as they strive to become family-centered in their work.

CHAPTER 10

APPLICATION TO SCHOOL-AGED CHILDREN
AND THEIR FAMILIES

When children enter school, roles and responsibilities within the family shift, and the family moves into a new phase of the childhood stage. Families with several children begin this change with the oldest child's advancement to school and enter a new phase when the child enters adolescence. Adolescence, the fourth family development stage (Carter & McGoldrick, 1989), continues until the family begins launching the oldest child. The developmental model delineates the beginning of a transition based on the age of the oldest child, but in many families, subsequent children necessitate that attention be paid to younger children that are following their unique developmental path.

FAMILY DEVELOPMENTAL FACTORS

The elementary school years tend to be less stressful for parents than the preschool years as children become increasingly independent, more facile in tending to their physical needs, and competent in peer relationships. In addition, the transition to school separates family members for increasingly longer periods of time during which the child develops personal competence. This relieves the parents from some of the intensity of their earlier caregiving duties.

When adolescence begins, many families become destabilized as new values, emotions, expectations, and personal styles are introduced into the family by the child and his or her peers. It may be impossible to "raise" teenagers. Perhaps, instead, they raise parents, and in the end the parents are wiser and more competent people as a result of all they have learned from their children. This chapter will focus on the early and later school years, including the adolescent transition. The case examples will describe family treatment with children having language, articulation, and phonological problems.

Parent-Child Interaction

Child-rearing is a process that requires the setting of appropriate boundaries while also encouraging the child's independence and personal decision-making within those boundaries. Infants are closely monitored, and the boundaries are tightly drawn around the mother, child, and other significant family members. The protection shown in these early years is necessary and appropriate. In well-functioning families, as the child matures, boundaries are gradually expanded until the individual reaches young adulthood and imposed family boundaries are no longer necessary since the individual is now able to make his own personal life decisions. The school years are critical to the child's successful development as personal competence, peer relationships, sibling relationships, and an identity that is separate from the family's is developed. Competent parents understand this and keep an appropriate balance between the imposition of boundaries and personal decision-making freedom. As the child matures, mistakes are made, lessons are learned, and successes are experienced. This gradual unfolding of life experiences interfaces with the child's developmental abilities and a mature, responsible adult eventually emerges often surprising his beleaguered parents.

Negotiating boundaries and personal freedom may be especially difficult for parents and children when special needs must be considered. The natural protectiveness of a mother for a preschool daughter who is deaf may persist into the school-age years as the difficult decisions about safe boundaries and personal freedom are established, changed, and re-established. Decisions relative to the restrictions placed on a ten-year-old with cerebral palsy must be made without impeding growth and maturation. The issues of adolescent sexuality, often problematic for parents whose children are "normal," must be confronted and explored as the child with special needs matures. The development of a personal identity, critical to every maturing individual, will not occur without trial and error, conflict, and parental sorrow as parents are once again reminded that their child's progress does not fall nicely into typical developmental norms. As each developmental milestone is approached, the parents must readjust their expectations to fit the capabilities of their child. This can be a complicated, difficult, *and* rewarding task.

Sibling Interaction

Sibling relationships take on new significance at this time. If the parents were sometimes overwhelmed by the needs of their child with a communicative disorder during the early years, they may now experience a sense of relief as he is enrolled in school and more free time is available to the adults in the family. This change may highlight the needs of typically developing children in the family who may not have received the attention they were due during their brother or sister's early years. An older sibling who takes on the role of the responsible child, may inadvertently become a third "parent" creating expectations well beyond reason when considered from the perspective of the older sibling's own developmental needs. Siblings often share the work associated with the added pressures of communicative delay and disability and, generally, benefit from the attitudes and abilities derived from these experiences. However, care must be taken to keep an appropriate balance between a sibling's involvement with a brother or sister who is communicatively disabled or delayed and that youngster's own developmental needs Family-Based Treatment offers an excellent opportunity to assist in this process while also benefiting the child with special needs.

We always invite the siblings of our speech-language clients to attend the family sessions. Younger siblings tend to attend every session while older siblings attend when the meetings do not conflict with their normal adolescent activities. The siblings typically are wonderful resources as we plan and develop treatment procedures. Their presence makes it possible to monitor sibling involvement so that it is balanced with developmental needs and parents' expectations and desires. A sister's or brother's fresh and unaffected desire to offer suggestions adds interest and fun to the family meetings. When sibling rivalry erupts, we can assess its impact on the communicative disorder, ask parents how they like to handle these conflicts, and normalize the disagreements so that siblings are encouraged to develop their own problem solving style within appropriate parentally established boundaries. Our experience clearly shows that school-age siblings appreciate being included in the treatment process. They gain, sometimes for the first time, an understanding of the communicative disorder and are appreciated members of the habilitative team. Some families that we have served in the past have contacted us to let us know that a sibling has decided to become a speech-language pathologist. One of these siblings told her mother that she had asked the director of her university program why she wasn't being taught about Family-Based Treatment! Perhaps an unintended consequence of a family-centered approach is wider public respect for the profession as parents and siblings become more aware of the usefulness of speech-language pathology services.

Peer Interaction

The importance of peer relationships is magnified for families having a child with disabilities. The strong desire of all people at every age level to develop meaningful friendships is particularly imposing during later childhood and early adolescence. The child who is developmentally disabled and who wants to have friends and relate well to peers may be rebuffed and forced to deal with the pain of rejection. Although not all children and adolescents with special needs are confronted with this problem, it is more common than for children who are developing normally. The mother of one of our adolescent clients tried, without success, to arrange a prom date for her daughter. She wanted her daughter to attend the prom with a boy having similar special needs. Her sensitive attention to this task failed, and the disappointment everyone experienced rippled through the speech-language treatment process.

Extended Family Interaction

Extended family members continue to be important to the client and his parents during the school years. Grandparents start to notice their own age-related changes, and adult children may have to shift their focus to the needs of their parents. This shift often happens while parents are simultaneously dealing with the behaviors of unpredictable adolescents. All family members change, as does the child with disability, as the family life cycle unfolds.

Families who have learned to acknowledge and deal with their differences related to raising a child with special needs will enjoy the support and continued help offered by grandparents, aunts, uncles, and other extended family members on whom the family has come to rely. Those who have not openly acknowledged and confronted these differences may experience increased tension relative to unsolicited advice and criticism from these and other relatives during the school-age years. In most cases, however, the speech-language clinician will find cooperative relationships between generations.

We are often surprised and always delighted to meet third and fourth generation family members that our families bring to family treatment sessions and are careful to include them in the process of the session. In these cases, we believe that the parents are aware of the importance of everyone understanding the efforts being made to create speech-language change and want to share this with their child's grandparents and great-grandparents. Involving three generations in treatment is not limited to a particular economic or social class. Most families seem to appreciate the support that can be offered by older generations. If conflict between generations, however, becomes evident as treatment proceeds this is a clue for us to ask the parents if they think it would be helpful to invite the grandparents to a meeting. When agreement to do this is reached, we are careful to structure the session so that the parents are supported in their parental role. This includes asking the parents to provide an explanation of the treatment that has been developed and our positively commenting on the parents' participation. Every time that we have arranged a session of this sort, the tension appears to be decreased between generations relative to the communicative disorder. The grandparent's love for their grandchild is accessed, and they are able to experience first hand the parental competence of their adult children as treatment procedures are described.

Siblings, extended family members, and even parents are not included in all sessions as the client matures into adolescence. Adolescent independence is reinforced when individual sessions are held with the permission of the parents and at the desire of the adolescent. This decision is reached jointly with the adolescent and his family members as partnership conversations lead to cooperative planning based upon an appreciation for the adolescent's maturational process. The adolescent may prefer such an arrangement and individual sessions are integrated into the Family-Based Treatment process.

CASE STUDIES

Articulation/Phonological Disorders

Errors in phoneme production are among those communicative problems that require the most structured and systematic approach to treatment. Treatment is characterized by small, orderly steps and consistent, discriminating use of reinforcement in order to shape the desired behavior. The effectiveness of interventions is obvious to the careful listener, and the behavior of the client clearly guides the clinician in the development of successive interventions. As we apply the Family-Based Treatment model to families having a member with one of these disorders, we are struck with how often the extent of generalization surpasses our expectations and with family members' ability to incorporate effective interventions into everyday activities. The latter is especially interesting since we traditionally view our procedures as requiring near-laboratory conditions in terms of the precision with which they should be introduced. Further, we do not usually think of phonology in terms of interactions as we do language and stuttering. This increases the challenge.

A very important principle that emerged as we used the model was to assign activities which the child would clearly be able to do. This means eliciting and practicing phonemes in contexts in which there is absolute certainty that the child and family can be successful nearly all the time. Family members are not asked to shape behavior as a speech-language pathologist would do or to make subtle or difficult distinctions between different productions of the same sound. Assignments are carefully developed to be isomorphic to each family's activities and resources. Clearly, if family members are to reinforce appropriate behavior, the behavior must be easily discernible in the course of natural interactions in noisy, and sometimes even chaotic, environments. Family members should be rewarded for their work just as the child is rewarded for new appropriate behavior. Assignments are idiosyncratic to each family and to each child and are based upon rewarding success for behavior that is near maximum in terms of effort possible in a natural setting. Further, goals must be clearly understood by family members, and the first goal is nearly always one which may be reached in several sessions. This is an important factor in empowering families and demonstrating that they can be successful. This same notion is a traditional principle that clinicians have applied to individual clients for many years. We merely adapt it to families. Within the context of the agreed-upon and achievable goal, each session consists of reviewing progress and searching for the maximum successful behavior possible. Still, the behavior has to be easily detectable to the family so that it can be rewarded appropriately.

Sometimes the child's immediate environment is other than the birth family. In this case, the system is defined to include the significant people who interact with the client on a daily basis. Tom, age thirteen, was a child like this. He had been removed from the home of his natural family and placed in a residential setting for boys whose families were not able to manage or care for them. The staff at the home was concerned about Tom's speech and made an appointment for an evaluation. Because Tom's records showed that he had been seen by the authors when he was younger, we were asked to re-evaluate him. Actually, we had seen him only one time when he was much younger. His family had been referred to us; we met for one session; but they were unable to continue as is often the case when parents are distressed and must struggle to meet their most basic needs. When we saw Tom six years later, he was a sullen, frightened, taciturn thirteen-year-old whose speech was unintelligible. He was accompanied by a representative of the home who obviously was concerned about him and attempted to interact with him. Tom did not reciprocate.

During this first session we listened to Tom's speech, but the majority of the time was spent attempting to define an appropriate interactive system with which to work. We were told that Tom's natural family was not available and could not be a part of that system. The representative who accompanied Tom neither knew him nor would be one who would interact with him other than to bring him to sessions. Because the residential setting was in a city some distance from the clinic in which we were working, the representative indicated that Tom would be limited to one session per week. At the same time, however, the staff who interacted with Tom wanted him to receive services. The representative thought that one counselor in particular interacted well with Tom and Tom with him. We ended the session with the understanding that the representative would speak with that counselor and attempt to arrange for him to accompany Tom to the next and subsequent weekly sessions.

Tom arrived the next week and was accompanied by a young man who identified himself as one of Tom's counselors. While Tom was far from effusive, there was an obvious difference in his manner, especially in response to the counselor. The counselor described Tom as being much like he was when he was young, and he believed that if Tom could develop a better self image, a natural result would be improved interactions with others. The counselor also described how Tom was teased and intimidated by two of the other boys. Tom agreed and named the boys. The counselor also discussed things he did in an attempt to help Tom. These included asking Tom to practice words that were especially difficult for him to say, having Tom practice saying the names of other counselors, and asking Tom to repeat the words "can of pop" when Tom requested this. Tom indicated that he was willing to do this and even liked practicing with the counselor. These activities were clear resources that could be elaborated upon and refined. An additional resource emerged with the counselor's description of his efforts to enhance Tom's place in the hierarchy of peers at the home. We agreed that the counselor would accompany Tom to sessions and that they would work together in the residential setting. We also agreed that he would garner the support of other counselors and even some of the boys who interacted with Tom. With this, the system was defined as Tom, the counselor, and the clinician. Subsystems, with which we would not come in contact, would include the counselor, Tom, and other counselors; the counselor, Tom, and other boys at the home; and various combinations of members of these groups.

Tom's speech was characterized by poor use of rhythm and intonation, deletion of final sounds, consistent use of a glottal stop for /g/ in prevocalic and intervocalic positions, omission of liquids or substitution of a plosive for a liquid, and many other inconsistent errors. Tom was stimulable for most sounds in isolation and in consonant-vowel syllables.

The counselor participated in the evaluation. The clinician administered the articulation test, did stimulability testing, and elicited other speech samples, but he also engaged the counselor in attempting to elicit correct sounds, syllables and words. The counselor was obviously comfortable in the situation and rewarded Tom well. He also found the idea of thinking about how sounds are produced fascinating and interesting. The counselor's genuine interest seemed to elicit interest from Tom. We viewed this as another resource. As we discussed goals, the counselor turned to Tom from time to time and asked him to repeat particular phrases, words, and sounds. Tom's counselor had noticed that the rhythm of Tom's speech was poor. The many articulation errors, including use of glottal stops, contributed to this. The counselor requested that whatever we did, it should be something with which Tom would be successful so that Tom's self-esteem might be improved.

We decided to delay setting a goal relative to a particular phoneme or phoneme group and, rather, have a general initial goal of improving the rhythm of Tom's speech and his awareness of the rhythm of speech. We found four, two and three-word phrases, which Tom could say perfectly. The assignment was for the counselor to elicit these from Tom in many different situations, making it as spontaneous and as much fun as possible, and to reward Tom appropriately. Tom agreed to participate in this activity and to cooperate fully. He was obviously pleased with how he sounded when he said these phrases and with his counselor's praise and pleasure when he did so. A second assignment was for the counselor to pay attention to other phrases that sounded perfect when Tom said them and to bring a list of these to the next session.

It should be noted that both assignments focused on positive features of Tom's ability. Since, as Wilcox (1989) points out, remediation inherently calls attention to deficits as the focus or topic of emphasis, it is important to assign interventions that capitalize on clients' abilities and strengths and to gradually nudge performance forward. We view this effort as part of our solution-focused approach. Families and clients who experience success and appropriate reward become empowered to undertake more and greater challenges. At the same time, they are less likely to be overcome by discouragement when an intervention is not successful.

Tom, his counselor, and a peer of Tom's from the home accompanied Tom to the third session. Both Tom and his counselor had enjoyed interjecting the phrases into natural practice situations, and the counselor had interested some of the other boys in aspects of speech production. This allied them with Tom in a new way. Not only were Tom's peers discouraged from teasing him, but Tom even gained new friends and supporters who appreciated Tom's new ability to "talk normally." The counselor had heard several additional phrases that Tom said well. We refined these during the session, had the counselor ask Tom to say them, and with Tom's permission, also engaged Tom's friend in this activity. All showed pleasure with Tom's "normal speech," and the assignment was continued for one more week.

At the fourth session, Tom noticed that what he did to sound normal was to exaggerate the movements of his mouth. We talked at some length about exactly what he felt he had been doing when his speech sounded good. Tom and the counselor had collaborated in developing a list of additional phrases that Tom could say perfectly. These were added to the list for Tom to practice using the techniques he now understood and was able to use intentionally. We also elicited a /g/ from Tom which had been difficult previously even though he was able to produce /k/. Tom and his counselor practiced Tom's production of /g/, and it was evident that even if Tom "lost" it, he and the counselor would be able to use the /k/ sound as a guide to "find" it again. A second assignment, in addition to practicing the phrases, was for Tom to practice producing /g/ (combined with a schwa) with his counselor. Reinforcing came so naturally for the counselor that he hardly had to be reminded that this was a very important part of the practice. A goal was set for Tom to be able to produce /g/ at will.

By the sixth session Tom was able to use the /g/ correctly in six words. He and his counselor had practiced increasing the speed with which he said these words and used the technique of combining them into artificial phrases with different rhythmical sequences. This was a method of combining the two assignments and using one to aid the other in a novel way. Both Tom and his counselor were rewarded for this innovation.

By this time Tom's speech intelligibility had improved. His interpersonal relations were markedly better. For the first time, he participated in events and initiated interaction with peers. He also walked and sat more deliberately, held his head so that he could look forward rather than down, and appropriately varied the expression on his face. Tom, his counselor, other staff at the home, and even many peers were pleased with these changes. Tom was reaping the rewards of his new interpersonal skills through intentional responses of others, but also in their unplanned, spontaneous reactions.

Treatment with Tom was terminated shortly thereafter when he moved out of the state. The interactive system that had become the unit of treatment was clearly different from the traditional family. Members of Tom's system responded creatively and resourcefully to our attempts to use their many resources. Assignments were isomorphic to the lifestyle of the residents and were created in a polyocular manner. This gave Tom's counselor a new and interesting way of thinking about speech. In all, we had seven sessions over a period of two months. Unfortunately, the details of Tom's move were not available to us, so we were not able to link with others who might be serving him in his new home. Tom's speech changed less than his pragmatics of interaction, but we all found great satisfaction with the results of our systemic treatment process.

When the problem is simply articulatory in nature, it might seem that family participation would be unnecessary. Yet in our experience, that is not necessarily the case. April, for example, was twelve years old and had a persistent lateral distortion of the "sh" sound. She had received speech-language services on an individual basis for five years. While other articulation errors were corrected during that time, the "sh" distortion persisted. In fact, the "sh" distortion had shown little change even after over one year of individual services focused on that sound alone. April's articulation was normal in all other respects.

April and her family were referred in hopes that family participation would make a difference. Since the problem was well defined and limited in scope, we agreed to having one parent involved in each session. We did, however, want both parents involved rather than have the same parent attend each session. April's mother participated in the first and subsequent sessions and, fortunately, after six sessions (and before the father was able to attend a session) April was using the "sh" sound accurately in conversational speech and was dismissed.

As with Tom, we wanted to build upon success and give assignments that could be carried out easily in the context of the family environment. At the first session the clinician was able to elicit a correct production of the "sh" sound in isolation, but April was not able to produce this with ease. It was clear that it was too early to assign April's mother to elicit the sound from April or for April to practice the sound. For this reason, the assignment given to the family at the first session was to let April *hear* the "sh" sound a lot but not to ask her to say it. Family members were to make the sound in isolation many times during the day in a playful way as they saw April and interacted with her. They were also to exaggerate the sound in words that came up in conversation with April and to intentionally say words containing the sound as they interacted with April. All of this was to be done in an enjoyable and friendly manner. No attempts were to be made to have April imitate family members' productions, and she was not to be asked to produce the sound or say words containing the sound.

When April and her mother arrived for the second session, they described how the assignment had been implemented. Both April and her mother agreed that no one had asked her to say anything. April, however, admitted that she had privately practiced the sound and that hearing it so much may have helped her. Clearly, something had helped her because she was able to find and produce the sound accurately and with ease. Her mother was surprised and pleased, and April received genuine acclaim from her.

From this point through the next four sessions, April was asked to let her family hear many productions of the sound (first in isolation and increasingly in syllables and words), and to practice increasing the speed with which she was able to read a list of words each containing an "sh" sound. In all cases, the interventions and practice were to be enjoyable and carried out during normal family activities, not during special times set aside for practice.

At the sixth session, April's mother and April both reported that the correct sound was part of April's natural articulatory repertoire. Both felt that no more sessions were necessary; the clinician agreed. One year later, April had maintained accurate use of the sound and had normal speech.

We are sure that the years of individual treatment that preceded our work with April laid the groundwork for rapid change. However, the involvement of family members (her mother and other family members recruited by her mother) completed the project. This change in the treatment model; the incorporation of interventions, practice, and reinforcement into everyday natural interactions; and the participation of the family in treatment seemed to be the factors that led to April's rapid success.

Language Disorders

Language is a complex issue, and although we advocate that families participate in the treatment of all types of language problems, it is understood that some aspects of language disorders will test the creative strategizing abilities of clinicians more than others. We have been very successful in helping a family effect change in its child's use of plurals, for example. Improving the same child's use of verb tense, however, was more difficult and frustrating. Plurals, as the child's parents pointed out, are easy; verb tense is complicated. Family interventions with plurals were easily made into enjoyable activities that could be carried out during and after meals, while watching television, and during the usual interactions of everyday life at home. All adults and older children in the family could easily make contributions because all understood the concept and could describe it. Interventions to improve verb tense were more challenging because more grammatical rules are involved, and more variations present themselves.

Ken's family helped him perfect his use of plurals. For example, Dad made up games such as having Ken guess how many pennies Dad had in his hand: "How many pennies do I have?" asked Dad. "I think you have one penny in your hand." "No, I have more than one penny. How many pennies do you think I have?" "I think you have four pennies." No, I have more than that, I have eight pennies. How many pennies did I have?" "You had eight pennies." "Good job, Ken!"

Ken's older brother also made up a game. He combined a number with an object to which Ken responded by changing plural to singular or singular to plural. For example, when Ken's brother said, "two ducks," Ken would respond, "one duck." This game was incorporated into mealtimes, when encountering one another in the house, in the car, etc. Both Ken and his brother enjoyed the game; Ken's brother especially liked to catch Ken "off guard" and surprise him with an intervention. Obviously, this was a playful family; different activities could be developed for families who spent more time reading books, engaging in physical activities, visiting grandparents, etc.

In our culture, the first natural response to a communicative disorder may be to ask the person questions. This seems to occur as a natural reaction independent of the problem or age of the person with the communicative difficulty. The second-most common response to children with language disorders may be to correct their speech. Since this is antithetical to building upon success and to reinforcing that success, it is important to creatively strategize with families in a manner that results in proactive, positive-outcome interventions built into family lifestyles.

Susan was a first grader whose correct use of past tense regular and irregular verbs was inconsistent. She lived with her mother, her mother's parents, and a nine-year-old sister. That group, along with the clinician, made up the interactive system. Everyone attended nearly all of the sessions, so access to the system was good.

All three adults had a tendency to ask Susan questions, to tell her what to say, and to correct grammatical errors they heard in Susan's spontaneous speech. Susan reacted to these attempts to help her by becoming sullen, by shouting (e.g., "don't tell me" or "no"), by withdrawing from the situation (e.g., crawling under the table, leaving the room, going to another part of the room and covering her ears with her hands), and/or by physically striking the "guilty" family member. These interactions seemed to be perpetuating the problem.

Family resources included a strong desire to help Susan improve her use of language, helpful grandparents who added to the number of adults who loved and cared for Susan, a strong positive relationship between Susan and her grandmother who enjoyed doing household chores together, and family members who enjoyed looking at books and reading with Susan. We focused our attention on these resources, incorporated them into our creative strategizing, and highlighted them in discussions with the family. Initially, we ignored those interactions that seemed to be perpetuating the problem, but when they did not change, we discussed them with the family. The use of counseling techniques was an important component of these discussions.

Assignments consisted of activities that built on family resources. We stressed that Susan should hear a lot of past tense verbs and be put in situations in which family members would use them for her to hear. Examples included emphasizing and even repeating short sentences and phrases with past tense verbs when looking at books; having grandmother review the housework she and Susan had done together emphasizing each past tense verb and repeating the phrase once or twice; and having Susan and her older sister review their day with one of the adults. When the use of questions, corrections, and requests to imitate did not subside, we gave an assignment to pay attention to the number of questions and corrections the adults used with Susan and to notice Susan's reaction to these. This was not intended to let the adults see how "bad" they were. Rather, the intent was to lay the groundwork for the adults to notice Susan's responses to other types of interventions and for an assignment to use techniques other than questioning and correcting. The earlier assignments, to let Susan hear her family members use and emphasize past tense verbs, was in preparation for asking them not to correct, ask questions, or request imitations. When family members are given assignments that include active interventions involving new ways of interacting, it may be easier for them to stop or reduce the interactions that perpetuate the problem because they are doing something new rather than merely trying not to do something.

After several sessions, family members began suggesting other activities which involved the use of past tense verbs. They had, for example, looked at family photographs with Susan. She enjoyed this, and since the photos involved past activities, past tense verbs flowed easily and naturally. The grandparents had developed a game in which one of them did an action. Then, together with Susan, the other grandparent described the action (e.g. you closed the door, you pushed your chair, etc.). At that point, we believed that we could assign them to repeat correctly phrases with past tense verbs that they heard Susan use incorrectly. They were not to call these to her attention, but merely to restate them correctly once or twice. Also, they were asked to reinforce those which they heard Susan use correctly. Another activity involved the adults audiotaping stories to which Susan listened, became familiar, and then retold. Still another activity was to read books that were familiar to Susan and to pause before saying some of the past tense verbs to let Susan say them and be rewarded for her successful use of the past tense.

Susan and her family enjoyed carrying out the assignments that we developed together. Interactions with Susan no longer consisted primarily of questions, corrections, and requests to imitate. In fact, these were rarely heard after five or six sessions. Susan's behavior improved along with the elimination of the interactions that she had come to dislike. Most importantly, Susan's use of past tense verbs improved, and correct usage became incorporated into her spontaneous speech.

SUMMARY

During the school years children gradually become less dependent on their parents. Sibling and peer relationships increase in importance, and as the child enters adolescence, issues associated with sexuality and impending adult independence begin to emerge. Families must learn how to allow the child to expand his boundaries while also maintaining appropriate personal control. Parental decision-making relative to the child with special needs continues as families learn to relate to schools and to the larger social service system.

Family-Based Treatment encourages developmentally appropriate sibling participation, parental and grandparental involvement, peer interaction, and the developing independence of the child or adolescent. When the child or adolescent is not living with immediate family members, other significant people from the child's environment may be successfully included in the treatment process.

CHAPTER 11

APPLICATION TO ADULTS AND THEIR FAMILIES

The launching process begins when children finish high school, move into the world of work and/or post secondary education, and begin to develop an independent lifestyle. The between families stage (Carter and McGoldrick, 1980) now commences for young adult children as intimate relationships are formed and decisions relating to sexuality, marriage, and childbearing are made. While these developmental changes are taking place, parents move on to relationship and career experiences that are often infused with a fresh sense of freedom.

FAMILY DEVELOPMENTAL FACTORS OF ADULTHOOD

Couples who are in their first marriage identify the launching stage as the most maritally satisfying of all the family developmental stages (Anderson, Russell & Schumm, 1983; Glenn, 1975; Rollins & Feldman, 1970). Solo parents gradually experience a lessening of financial and care-giving responsibility and may, for the first time in many years, have time to attend fully to their own adult needs. The launching stage is filled with numerous family exits and entrances as people leave, return, and leave again often accompanied by friends, partners, wives or husbands, and grandchildren. The parental expectation that the launching process will be smooth and brief is usually unfulfilled, particularly when children participate in post-secondary education or protracted career exploration requiring financial support well beyond age twenty-one, the usual age of independence. Families with several children may be launching one or more children while also dealing with school-aged and adolescent offspring. Launching interfaces with the later years stage as grandparents and great-grandparents begin to require additional attention and support. The complexities and challenges of family life continue, often accompanied by unanticipated events such as illness, divorcing children who return home, and grandparental child-care responsibilities.

When all children are launched, parents enter their child-free years and begin planning for retirement. As parents (grandparents) approach age 65, the family begins its last stage, the later years. Advancements in medical care allow people to live longer, the quality of life has improved for most older families, and many people remain active well into their eighth and ninth decades (Vander Zanden, 1989). Furthermore, variations in temperament, cognitive ability, physical stamina, and social interests between people of similar ages create a mosaic of behavior that is decidedly heterogeneous. For example, two normal seventy-five-year-olds will vary in motor, cognitive and social ability to a much greater extent than will two adolescents. Our seventeen-year-old son noted this variation as he admired the strength and stamina of a seventy-seven-year-old man who was part of a 400 mile, week-long bicycle tour across the state of Iowa. Our son was impressed by the gentleman's physical ability as well as by his "old-fashioned" single speed bicycle, quite unlike the high tech models ridden by many of the adolescent, young adult, and middle-aged adult participants. Almost any healthy seventeen-year-old could manage such a tour; fewer seventy-seven-year-olds could survive this arduous journey. Sensitivity to this tremendous variation in individual ability and circumstance must be integrated into the speech-language pathologist's clinical skills repertoire when working with older adults.

Family life during the launching and moving on stage, as well as during the later years, is characterized by many interwoven events. The spiraling generations weave a tapestry of complex relationships that change with each new generation yet show intricately-related patterns that are intergenerationally connected as grandchildren and great-grandchildren are born and new generations are formed. The "last" stage is final for one part of the generational spiral but not for the family system since every stage of the life cycle is interrelated to every other stage. The interconnectedness of the family is powerfully experienced during these "last" two stages of the family life cycle. In this chapter we will review the impact of disability on these stages and describe family involvement in the treatment of communicative disorders associated with aphasia and mental retardation.

Shifting Parent-Young Adult Interaction

Independence stands out as a major goal to be achieved during the launching stage of the family life cycle. This goal includes the physical independence experienced when a child establishes an apartment, moves to a college dormitory, or continues to live at home (with fewer restrictions than were imposed previously) while they also prepare for financial independence. Sooner or later, personal mastery of career skills appropriate to the early adult years occurs, and financial credibility is established, thus freeing parents of the financial burdens of the early launching stage. Intimate relationships are explored and developed, and the young adult begins to make decisions that may or may not correspond to the decisions made by the parental generation during their early adult years.

Concurrently, parents become independent of child-rearing responsibilities, and new opportunities for their own personal, career, and relationship development are created. A mutual separation between parents and young adult children occurs and is experienced as exciting, challenging, and perhaps foreboding as the young person succeeds, flounders, reorganizes, and moves on, eventually establishing complete physical, career, and financial independence. In some families, parents are confronted with a returning launched adult who is going through a divorce, has lost his or her job, or requires special care related to an unexpected problem such as alcoholism. Unanticipated developmental disruptions increase family stress and create dilemmas that require creative problem solving skills.

Developmental disability has a powerful impact on emerging independence. Some families in which a young adult has a developmental disability will traverse the launching transition with the same equanimity found in most other families and will, after four or five years, be pleased and sometimes surprised to discover that their child has moved successfully into adult independence. This independence may take a different form from that of a person who is nondisabled but is, nonetheless, achieved. Other families may not be able to achieve independence for themselves and their adult child for financial reasons or because of the severity of the disability.

Two family issues may be particularly evident to the speech-language pathologist during this transition. First, an accident or illness may create a permanent disability and serious, unexpected individual and family developmental disruption. Second, family disruption may appear to be evident in the parent-child relationship of the young adult who has been disabled since childhood as adult independence becomes an issue. Both of these issues may seem to create transitional upheaval. Let us now turn our attention to the developmental concerns related to each of these issues.

Unexpected Illness or Accident

The sudden disruption of an accident or illness pulls the family back into the life of the young adult just as he or she has begun or just completed the transition to adulthood. Head injury, for example, can occur at any time in the life cycle, but the incidence is highest for males between fifteen and thirty-five and peaks in the fifteen to twenty-four-year-old range (Rollin, 1987). The family's energy is immediately focused on the preservation of life. The brief sense of elation that is experienced when life is assured is followed by days, months, years, and sometimes a lifetime of concern for the quality of life that their loved one might achieve (DePompei, 1987). Furthermore, variations in complications, ranging from minor to major, make each case unique and require clinician sensitivity to the idiosyncratic responses of the client and his family members as effects are assessed and treated.

Attention to intergenerational issues is imperative. If a person who is head-injured is married with young children, the young family is irrevocably changed as spouse and children attempt to accommodate to their "new" family member. If the young adult is not married or if divorce occurs following the injury, aging parents must often abandon their newly acquired freedom and return to a caregiving role. As the clinician involves these family members in the treatment process, attention to their resources as well as the stressors that are impacting each family member is essential to the effective application of the Family- Based Treatment model. Families that had a workable problem-solving style premorbidly will access these intact resources and, in spite of their pain, begin to accommodate to their changed family member. Families that were conflicted and chaotic premorbidly will continue to show those same behaviors and will surely tax the clinician's creative strategizing abilities.

Developmental Disability

Families that have been raising their child with a disability since childhood face different challenges. One cannot help empathizing with the pain and grief of the family with a newly injured family member. On the other hand, families that have been dealing with disability for years are often expected to have adjusted to the problem and may not elicit empathy from the professional community. Nevertheless, it is critical for the clinician to remember that developmental transitions usually remind the family, once again, that their loved one is not "typical" and that they now have another set of issues with which to deal. What kind of job, if any, will the emerging adult be able to secure? How will he/she deal with relationships and sexuality? Is independent living possible, and, if so, how much involvement should parents have? What will happen when the support systems that are readily available until age twenty-one are no longer accessible? What will happen when parents, if they are the caregivers, become ill and/or too old to care for their adult family member? And, even though the young adult and his/her parents may be well aware that handicaps are made, not born, what will happen when parents are no longer available to smooth over the anguish created by a society that has not yet learned this important fact? These and other questions may disrupt the family of the young adult as the launching years begin.

The clinician must deal with yet another factor that compounds the treatment problems associated with launching. Many families have spent twenty years or more struggling to maintain their appropriate role as parents of their child. A major part of this struggle has taken place in the offices and classrooms of the specialists that have served their child. They have heard the message from some of these professionals: "You are a problem and are not welcome. Your child would be doing well if it weren't for your over-involvement with him." Professionals don't actually say this, of course, but parents may believe they hear this unfortunate message. Each professional encounter has added another layer of protection to the parent-child dyad unless the family was fortunate, early on, to have encountered a professional who helped empower the parents in their appropriate role. The clinician that wants to involve the family in treatment during the launching phase may experience this parental protection as hostility and will need to employ reflective listening and an extra measure of respect before family members can begin to trust that their participation is really desired. Family members that appear to be "overprotective" must be enlisted on the team so that their love for their young adults is accessed and their consultative expertise is effectively utilized for change.

The young adult who is moving toward independence will do so more successfully if family support and assistance are integral parts of the process. An understanding of the launching stage of family development as it occurs for all families and as it impacts families experiencing disability will help the clinician involve the family in the assessment and treatment of speech language change.

Aging Parent-Adult Interaction

During the later years stage, family interaction changes as the aging process begins to affect marital relationships, physical abilities, and the financial stability of the aging family member. The later years are a time of continuing growth and change for many individuals while steady decline and physical difficulties characterize the lives of others. Death marks the final exit of family members from the intergenerational spiral just as birth marked the individual's entrance into the family. Death, however, does not necessarily eliminate the influence of the individual who has had a unique impact on the family as it has evolved over time.

Changing marital relationships impact older adults in a number of ways. Retirement creates shifts in relationships that are easily accommodated by couples who enjoy role flexibility. These couples look forward to their retirement years and anticipate increased freedom to enjoy one another, leisure activities, and in some cases a new career. Couples who are not accustomed to role flexibility will experience a period of adjustment when retirement occurs if the retired person feels bereft of responsibility while the partner feels that her territory has been invaded by an ever-present spouse. When retirement plans are destroyed by a debilitating stroke, heart attack, or other disease, a severe developmental disruption occurs. When a spouse dies, the associated stress experienced by his life-long partner is the most serious of any stressor of the later years (McCubbin & Dahl, 1985).

Physical changes that are a natural part of aging vary in impact for older adults, but each person becomes aware of a gradual decline in physical abilities. Most adjust quite easily to these normal body changes while others require frequent medical intervention.

Financial stability is critical to successful aging, but the widening gap between those who are financially stable and those whose means are sparse reflects the economic disparity evident in the wider culture. When finances are inadequate and family financial support is not available, the older adult is unable to age gracefully. Poverty and isolation are serious extenuating circumstances for many elderly persons, particularly females who outlive their male peers. The clinician is likely to encounter people from a variety of life circumstances, all of whom are dealing with the disabling effects of a communicative disorder.

Any or all of the changes during the later years activate the younger generations who must now join in the decision-making process relative to their older family members. Spouses, adult children and their spouses, grandchildren, brothers, and sisters are essential members of the habilitative team as plans are made to maximize communicative competence. In the unfortunate event that the older adult has no family members available to participate in treatment, friends, acquaintances, and professional staff in long-term care facilities can be enlisted to help develop an understanding of functional language needs and to participate in the development of appropriate interventions.

When it is clear that speech-language treatment will not enhance the well-being of the aging adult and that change is not realistically possible, the ethical clinician will inform the family or caregiving institution of this fact and offer suggestions for alternative activities that may make the loved ones last months as comfortable as possible.

The later years stage of the family life cycle continue to be filled with complex changes that interface with the ever-evolving changes experienced by other family members. The interactive abilities of family members can be accessed, supported, and altered to assist in the enhancement of communicative strategies as speech-language-hearing treatment occurs.

LAUNCHING AND LATER YEARS CASE STUDIES

Speech-Language Problems Associated with Mental Retardation

The launching transition can be very stressful for the individual and family of the person who is mentally retarded. The grieving process may be reawakened as the family is confronted with a new set of issues. All families are faced with new tasks during the launching stage, but usually with the knowledge that the child's full independence is possible and with the expectation that it will be achieved. However, the parents of a young adult who is mentally retarded are likely to experience stress and isolation during the launching transition that is second only to that experienced at the time of the original diagnosis (Wikler, et al., 1983; Suelzle & Keenan, 1981).

Until now, school placement and support had been a major focus of the family, and the loss of this management assistance can be a difficult and seemingly insurmountable challenge for many parents (Long, 1990). In addition, the adult social service system presents a confusing array of possibilities that the family may not understand or know how to access, and family members must take on the unfamiliar role of case manager for their adult child. If they have been encouraged in this role since their child's early years, they will be accustomed to problem solving and will have the confidence and ability to meet the task at hand. If their parental role has been gradually usurped by well-meaning professionals, they are likely to flounder precariously as this management task is handed over to them. The family's search for services or a rehabilitation counselor's referral may bring the launching individual and family to the speech-language pathologist's door.

Mrs. Stevens, Bob's mother, called the speech-language clinician soon after her son's twenty-third birthday. Bob had just been accepted by a sheltered workshop following a vocational rehabilitation assessment and was having difficulty following directions and communicating with supervisors and co-workers. The workshop supervisor suggested that speech-language treatment might facilitate

Bob's communicative competence and help him integrate into the work situation.

Mrs. Stevens said that she didn't know exactly why the referral had been made because she understood Bob perfectly and wondered aloud if the people at the workshop were treating her son fairly. The clinician suggested that since the mother was able to communicate successfully with her son, it would be very helpful if she could accompany him to the first session. Mother readily agreed.

During the telephone convening conversation, the clinician learned that Bob was an adult with mental retardation, living at home with his mother and father, and that his two older sisters were launched and lived some distance from the parental home. The clinician asked Mrs. Stevens to invite her husband to accompany her and Bob to the session. She replied that he would probably come but would not say much because he usually left these things up to her. Appreciation was expressed to Mrs. Stevens for inviting her husband, and she was assured that it was fine if her husband did not want to talk much and that he probably would not speak unless he had something important to share. It was hoped that this statement would relieve Mrs. Stevens of the worry that her "quiet" husband would be pressured into contributing when he was unwilling to do so. Since Mr. Stevens was recently retired and Mrs. Stevens was a homemaker, a daytime appointment was arranged immediately following the end of Bob's work day.

The family arrived at the appointed time. Bob, a large gregarious man, greeted the clinician with an affable smile and immediately reached out to shake the clinician's hand. The clinician introduced herself, chatted a bit, and asked Bob to introduce her to his parents. This act immediately underscored Bob's status as an emerging adult who would be the primary focus of the clinician's work while simultaneously indicating the importance of his parents as consultants to the treatment process. Mom smiled pleasantly and following her introduction to the clinician instructed Bob to remove his jacket because "It's hot in here." Bob readily complied and the clinician led the family to the treatment room where the introductions were completed. Mr. Stevens, a quiet person possessing the same size and apparent physical strength of his son, looked glum and a bit unhappy as he seated himself in the room. His quiet demeanor was a powerful contrast to the animated discussion taking place between Mrs. Stevens and Bob as they discussed the temperature of the room and the advisability of wearing jackets and coats.

The clinician noted to herself that Bob was wearing a hearing aid, a fact that she had failed to learn during the initial telephone conversation. She also noted that Bob's speech was characterized by difficulty with sibilant sounds and that his rapid rate of speech added to his unintelligibility.

The family interview and the accompanying spontaneous enactments clearly underscored Mrs. Stevens' belief that she understood Bob perfectly. The clinician was able to understand most of Bob's utterances and whenever she appeared to be somewhat quizzical, Mrs. Stevens willingly and readily interpreted. Each time this happened, Bob was asked if his mother's interpretation was correct and only once did he have to alter what she had said. No overt communication was observed between Mr. Stevens and his son.

Bob was asked to read words and sentences to assess his articulation further. As Mr. Stevens observed this process, his unhappy facial expression was replaced by a look of curiosity and amusement. The clinician hypothesized that this may have been one of the few times that he had participated in a visit to a professional's office relative to his son's habilitative program.

The clinician explained her findings as she learned the characteristics of Bob's speech. She discussed the fact that he had a mild, inconsistent hypernasality; a number of inconsistent errors on consonants; and a consistent oral distortion of sibilant sounds, most notably /s/. Mrs. Stevens reiterated that she understood Bob perfectly, and the clinician responded that this was absolutely true, but apparently people who did not know Bob as well as she did had some difficulty communicating with him. Mr. Stevens then spoke for the first time saying that, "Even people who know him well have trouble." The clinician asked if that was sometimes the case for him, and he replied, "Yes." Mrs. Stevens offered the suggestion that treatment might be good so that other people could understand him, but that they would also have to try a little harder and learn to be more patient with Bob. The clinician responded by asserting that this was a good point and that a meeting with the people at the workshop might facilitate a better understanding of the difficulties experienced in that setting. Mrs. Stevens was assured that she would also be part of the meeting, as would Bob, and she offered to try to schedule a meeting.

Data gathering continued as the clinician questioned Bob about his hearing loss and the effects of this on his communication with other people. He said that he often had difficulty understanding other people, particularly when the TV was on. In a quiet room during face-to-face contact, he "can understand everything." The clinician asked Bob to get an audiological evaluation and gave him instructions for making the appointment. Mr. Stevens said that he would see that Bob had transportation to the appointment.

Tentative times for a workshop meeting were discussed, exchange of information forms signed, and the first session ended. The clinician noted that Mr. Stevens seemed relaxed and less glum than at the start of the session and asked him if he too would be interested in attending a meeting at the sheltered workshop. His reply, "I suppose so," was viewed as positive, and the family departed the first session.

The results of the audiological examination revealed a moderate-to-severe sensorineural loss for the right ear and a profound hearing loss in the left ear. The hearing aid worn in the right ear produced a speech reception threshold at 20 dB HL and a speech discrimination score of 76 percent.

At the beginning of the second session, the clinician reaffirmed Mrs. Stevens' ability to communicate effectively with her son and asked the parents if they were willing to go along with Bob's desire for improvement since this might help him communicate with his peers in his new job situation. Mr. and Mrs. Stevens agreed and said that a meeting had been arranged at the sheltered workshop to further assess Bob's communicative difficulties.

Speech-language treatment included the development of communication strategies such as slower speech, exaggerated articulation, increased effort, and increased pitch as well as attempts to improve his production of specific consonants. Bob explained to his father that he could understand him better if they faced each other when they talked and if Dad would "SPEAK UP." The clinician conducted the sessions as she would have conducted individual sessions but with the parents present and participating as they wished. Both Mr. and Mrs. Stevens became increasingly comfortable asking questions and making suggestions. A turning point seemed to occur when Mr. Stevens suggested that he and Bob could probably talk better if the TV were turned off.

The network meeting at the sheltered workshop identified the problems Bob had communicating with peers when the environment was noisy, and the decision was made to move him to a job in a quieter environment. There he would associate with only two other people and would be less overwhelmed as he attempted to slow his rate of speech and implement his newly acquired articulation strategies. Everyone present was asked to pay attention to Bob's communication and to encourage Bob as he made an effort to communicate more effectively. The friendly, cooperative style shown by everyone at the meeting pleased Bob and his parents.

Treatment continued for six months. At the end of the second month, Mr. and Mrs. Stevens felt that they understood what was going on and decided to go out for coffee while Bob was in his session. This appropriate differentiation underscored Bob's independence from his parents. The parents felt that they didn't need to be "watching over him every minute" since he was already twenty-three years old.

Maximum change occurred as a result of Bob's efforts, the cooperation of his parents, and the reinforcement received from the staff of the sheltered workshop. Mrs. Stevens remarked that even she found it easier to talk to her son. Treatment terminated with the understanding that Bob would call the clinician if he decided he needed further help. His speech was not perfect, but significant changes had occurred. He was interacting more effectively with his father and had received the "Worker of the Month" award at the sheltered workshop.

Treatment Related To Aphasia

Clients who seek the services of a speech-language pathologist for difficulties related to aphasia can achieve benefits from family involvement. Managed care now limits the dollars that are available for speech-language services to these clients thus limiting the number of sessions that can be provided in in-patient as well as out-patient facilities. Partnerships with the client and family members make it possible to provide the "best possible" treatment in these cases by incorporating family members into the treatment process (Burns, 1996).

This serves two goals: first, the patient can receive communication interactive practice within the context of his or her relationships in his living situation. This provides the potential for active treatment to continue during the patient's normal daily activities. Second, the patient can focus on functional goals that meet both personal communicative needs and those important within his or her relationships. The ability to target goals of interest to both the family and the patient provides an added incentive to actively participate in all aspects of the speech rehabilitation process. (Burns, 1996, pp. 116)

Clients' family members may be ready and able to participate in treatment or, they may be unavailable due to distance or other factors. Burns has included clients' work colleagues, close friends, a "sister" of a nun in a convent, and primary caretakers as well as family members in family-based treatment sessions, while also documenting client change for managed care purposes. (Burns, 1996).

In other cases, clinicians who work systemically may be called upon by families for one or two-session consultations. Families who request this are not seeking assessment and treatment in the usual sense but want the speech-language pathologist's opinion about a communicative problem and/or suggestions for ways to improve interaction with a family member having a communicative disorder. Termination of services is expected after the number of agreed-upon sessions has been completed.

A consultation session was requested by the family of Mrs. Alban, an 85-year- old woman who lived in a nursing home. Her family included three adult children and their spouses. All lived within fifty miles of the nursing home and visited her on a regular basis. The clinician was contacted by one of the adult children and asked to meet with Mrs. Alban and her family in the nursing home to discuss how communication with her could be enhanced. Mrs. Alban's family believed that she wanted to interact with them but could not "move her mouth correctly" to do so.

We met with Mrs. Alban and her family in the sunroom of the nursing home. Family members present included her two daughters and her son and his wife. Mrs. Alban was in a wheel chair repeating, "wishy-wishy" in a quiet voice looking at nothing or no one in particular. We watched as family members spoke with her and observed that nearly every interaction was a question (e.g., Do you know who's here? Who am I, Mom? Did you remember to take your pill? What day is it? Did you have breakfast? What did you eat? Did you eat it all? Were you able to eat today? Did the nurses help you? Do you know where we are?) or commands (e.g., C'mon Mom, you've got to try. Try my name; say Mike. Today is Monday; you say it. Say Monday, Mom. Look at me; watch my mouth. Watch!).

After observing the attempts of family members to interact with Mrs. Alban, we made a special point of neither asking questions nor giving commands as we initially spoke with her. Rather, we attempted to make only statements. Mrs. Alban did not actually respond to these any differently than she did to the questions and commands of her children. In fact, if anything, she seemed more pleased to hear her children's voices than ours.

We listened as family members gave their perspective of the problem. They sensed the gravity of the problem even though they continued to use terms implying that their mother's communicative ability would improve. As we talked more and observed one another interact with Mrs. Alban, it became clear that change in her expressive communicative behavior was not a realistic goal. We began asking for information about the adult children's common family as they were growing up, their mother's interests, their father's characteristics, and their mother's role in the family. What evolved was a mini-history of the family with each adult child being eager to relay interactions that he or she had had with mother. They described their mother as a key person in the home as they were growing up and one who had made most of the decisions, done most of the disciplining, and who was primarily responsible for the care of the children. At this point we returned to our discussion of the severity of Mrs. Alban's communication problem. We suggested that they talk about childhood and family experiences as they interact with their mother in order to remind her, to the extent possible, of past events and to provide communicative input that she might enjoy. We framed the latter suggestion in terms of the life review (Lewis & Butler, 1974) that is very meaningful when done by and with older persons as they near the end of life. We pointed out that their mother responded more positively to their voices than she did to ours and that if they were to speak slowly while touching her hand or arm (which they had already been doing) she might appreciate these memories more than attempts to orient her and "demonstrate" her understanding.

The consultation session lasted one and one-half hours. The family members expressed appreciation for our help and seemed satisfied that they were doing all that they could for their mother. A follow-up session was scheduled to be held in two months.

Consultation sessions can also be conducted with staff at adult living facilities. These systemic consultations can lead to changes in the client's living situation that facilitate independent living as well as a higher quality of life. When working with aging persons whose communication is severely disordered, a family/staff consultation session is likely to help those who interact with the client establish communication strategies that may make the later years more comfortable for their family member. The aging person will also benefit from the loving concern offered by the people who mean the most to him.

SUMMARY

Significant developmental changes occur during the adult years. The launching family must adjust to their emerging young-adult member who is establishing independence. When injury or illness disrupts this process, the impact on the family is often severe. Families must also accommodate to their young-adult member who has been developmentally disabled since childhood as his/her role in the larger society is defined.

Older family members often enjoy active and productive lives and are supportive members of their children and grandchildren's treatment teams. Other aging persons may be forced to deal with illness and disability. Family support is critical to the well-being of these individuals and the speech-language pathologist should enlist the family's help as treatment is planned and implemented. When family members are unavailable, friends and professional staff may be recruited to provide communication reinforcement in the older person's natural context.

CHAPTER 12

WORKING WITH CHALLENGING
FAMILY SITUATIONS

In this chapter we will discuss several of the challenging family situations that we have encountered in our Family-Based Treatment practice. We use the word "challenging" rather than "problem" or "difficult" because a "challenging situation" calls for concentration, creativity and a desire to do something different; this reframe helps us think and act in a solution-focused way. We use the phrase "family situation" rather than "family" to help us shift from labeling behaviors to identifying interactive patterns. We are interested in the systemic interactions that surround the situation, including our participation in the process, rather than in labeling the family members in a negative way. Further, we recognize that there are many "truths" associated with every challenging experience and that the family might describe the situation quite differently than we do; their experience is as valid as ours and we strive to be empathically curious about their understanding of the situation.

Each clinician's experience is also different from ours, and the reader may be surprised that we have been challenged by these particular situations or may wonder why situations that she has experienced have not been included. Therefore, a word of explanation is in order; we will discuss the situations that we *personally* have experienced and will not attempt to address those that we have not experienced. The cases have been sufficiently disguised to protect the identity of the families, but all are accurate examples of our response to these situations. We hope that our descriptions will help the reader to create her own solutions to the challenges that she experiences in her interaction with families. The chapter is divided into three sections: the self of the clinician, family-clinician differences, and internal family difficulties.

THE SELF OF THE CLINICIAN

There are some personal strategies that can be developed to make it easier for a clinician to work with challenging family situations. Some of these are the following: cultivate patience, respect difference, use counseling techniques, develop clear boundaries, and connect with supportive colleagues.

Cultivate Patience

Justin's parents were embroiled in a contentious divorce. Nevertheless, they were both willing to participate in speech-language services because they were concerned about their son's lagging language development and unintelligible speech. The clinician felt challenged by the animosity that accompanied Justin and his parents to their sessions and wondered what possessed her to work systemically with this family; it would have been so much easier to meet with Justin alone in order to avoid his parent's conflict. The clinician remained patient, however, remembering that change is occurring all the time, that Justin was profoundly affected by his parent's divorce, and that the child would surely benefit from his parent's positive involvement in creating speech language change. Later, the clinician's patience paid off as she developed a strong relationship with the two most important people in Justin's life. Both parents, though conflicted, were eager to provide the speech-language stimulation that Justin needed. Details of Justin's situation will be described later in this chapter.

Respect Difference

Jennifer, Angela's mother, was young; she was 16 years old when Angela was born and only 19 when she came to her first Family-Based Treatment session. Jennifer's mother and grandmother, with whom she lived, also attended the session. All were involved in caring for Angela and concerned that, at age three, Angela spoke few words. All three women repeatedly asked Angela questions which she did not answer. Instead Angela responded with loud "no's" and frequent temper tantrums. The three parents then disciplined her with lectures (which Angela clearly did not understand) and discussed the child in derogatory terms. The clinician remembered that he must be patient. If he alienated Angela's parents they

would not want to continue working with him, and he would have no opportunity to introduce other ways of interacting. He also recognized that parenting styles are bound to intergenerational cultural norms that are long-
standing and firmly established. As a speech-language pathologist and as a
parent, he knew that he would not treat the child in this way, but he also
knew that a parenting lecture would not help him join with the family. He
chose to listen carefully to their concerns and pay attention to their attempts
to help. He did this intending to uncover resources that could be activated for
speech language change. Patience (in full measure) and respect for difference helped him work successfully with this case. Details about Angela's
family situation will be described later in this chapter.

Use Counseling Techniques

Peter, a child with Down syndrome, was a member of a large, loving family. The clinician enjoyed working with Peter and his family because
they quickly became full partners in treatment and responded positively to
isomorphic suggestions. Peter, at age five, was making excellent progress
and would soon be mainstreamed into kindergarten. The clinician was surprised and confused when the parents suddenly expressed disappointment
with their child's progress and questioned the clinician about the possibility
of initiating more tests. Instead of responding defensively, the clinician
decided to clarify and reflect the parents' concerns. As he listened, he
learned that Peter's mother, Mary Jo, had spent the week visiting area
schools in order to make an informed decision about Peter's kindergarten
placement. In the process, Mary Jo had transitioned into a grieving cycle and
was once again grieving the loss of the dream (see Chapter 8). The clinician
continued to listen and then offered to do some additional testing. Mary Jo
said that she didn't want more testing after all, and the family shifted the
conversation to the business of communicating with Peter. Counseling techniques were woven into the treatment process in order to show respect and
understanding for the family's re-emerging grief.

Develop Clear Boundaries

A clinician was working with several families whose children had
been diagnosed on the autism spectrum. She knew, from experience, that
grieving (see Chapter 8) would accompany most of the families to their sessions. Tracy's parents had suspected for some time that something was seriously different about their daughter and were, in one sense, relieved to final-

ly have a diagnosis. This gave them the opportunity to search out more information on the internet, from other parents, and from the clinician herself.

Tracy's mother, Connie, called the clinician frequently after receiving her daughter's diagnosis, and the clinician patiently answered Connie's questions while also reflecting the mother's grief and disappointment. One phone call came at a time when the clinician was unable to spend more than two minutes conversing. The clinician politely and empathically used an I-statement (see Chapter 8), and Connie respectfully ended the conversation. The clinician knew that she must respect her own boundaries in order to continue to enjoy her challenging work. Further, in all of her work, the clinician drew clear boundaries around her personal life with her own family; she remembered to leave her concerns about work at the office in order to enjoy leisure time with friends and loved ones. Challenging families can empty a clinician's personal reserves if she fails to draw clear boundaries in order to protect her personal and professional life.

Connect with Supportive Colleagues

Jack's parents requested services that the clinician could not provide due to policies that had been established by her workplace. The clinician met with Jack and his family infrequently and did not feel well-joined with them but, nevertheless, knew that she must tell them that she could not provide the specific services they wanted. She prepared for the meeting by identifying alternative resources that the family could explore but was wary about talking with the parents as they were very assertive about their child's needs. The parents showed anger when the clinician told them that she would not be able to provide the services they wanted and threatened to sue the organization for which she worked. She recognized that their feelings were associated with Jack's diagnosis as well as with the news that the services requested could not be provided, but this did not make the situation any easier. The clinician reflected the parents' anger, expressed her regret that she could not provide the services requested, and shared the resources that she had identified. Nevertheless, she felt "drained" by the end of the meeting and wondered why she ever decided to work with families in the first place!

Karl Whitaker, a well-known family therapist, once said that every family therapist needs a cuddle group. We think he meant that those of us who work with challenging family situations need supportive colleagues to sustain us when our work becomes overwhelming. In this case, the clinician sought out a colleague who understood the context in which the therapist worked and was able to listen empathically to the clinician's feelings about her recent contact with Jack's family. Supportive colleagues are essential to the clinician's well-being when she is working with challenging family situations.

RESPONDING TO FAMILY-CLINICIAN DIFFERENCES

Forty years of psychotherapy outcome research indicates that the most important factor in successful treatment occurs outside the context of therapy (Duncan, Miller and Hubble, 1997). Duncan and his colleagues, who are doing pioneering work with cases that have been identified as "impossible," call these factors extratherapeutic. In other words, the client's perception of the problem and the client's expectations for treatment influence outcome more than any other single factor. Interestingly, this is a factor over which the therapist has no control. If she is to be successful in working with "impossible" cases, she must be willing and able to fully understand the client's reality and to suggest changes that fit with that reality. The second most important factor in successful treatment, according to Duncan's research, is associated with therapeutic relationship factors. That is, when the client experiences the therapist as caring, concerned, empathic and non-judgmental treatment is more likely to be successful than if those factors are not present. To us this means that if the speech-language clinician wants to work successfully with difficult family situations, she must strive to understand the family's reality and the environmental factors that contribute to that reality while also creating a caring, respectful partnership. This is *not* done to try to change the family's reality but rather to understand it so that suggestions can be created that make sense to the family and help them get what they want from treatment.

The shifts in thinking that are described in chapter one, isomorphic suggestions that are described in chapter five, the counseling techniques that are described in chapter eight, and the principles of family-centered treatment as described in chapter nine, fit well with the understanding that the family's reality is key to successful treatment partnerships. When the clinician is dealing with challenging family situations, the principles described in these chapters should be followed if effective treatment is to occur. Most importantly, change will not occur without respect for the family's view which can be quite *different* from the clinician's view. We believe that colliding differences create most of the challenging situations that speech-language-hearing professionals encounter.

Economic Differences

Speech-language pathologists and audiologists do not live in poverty. Some of our clients, however, experience the daily ravages of poverty. Graduate students and I (Jim) have done many home visits as part of an early intervention training grant project. Some of the homes we visited were very dirty; cockroaches scurried across the floor; chairs were sticky and covered with grime. In one case, a young single mother lived in such a place. She could not afford dental care, and as we were conversing, her gums bled, coloring her teeth red. She seemed to be embarrassed about her situation and said that this was not the life she wanted for her or her family. She explained that the apartment in which she lived was not cared for by the landlord; the bathtub faucet had been broken for two weeks; the windows did not close properly; she did not have a phone; and, when she told the manager of the complex about these problems, he "put me off" with promises that were not kept. Nevertheless, she cared deeply for her children even in the midst of her substandard living situation. A member of the early intervention team helped connect her to appropriate community services who resettled her into better housing. Dental care was also arranged. As these services were put in place she was more able to focus on the speech-language needs of her son. She seemed to welcome our visits as we did not criticize or avoid her situation (washable pants helped with this) but, instead, enjoyed being with her and helped her find services to relieve some of the effects of poverty.

Ethnic/Cultural Differences

The ethnicity of our client families is often different from ours, and we work with many families whose first language is not English. We cannot work with children from these families without parental participation as they must help us with the challenges that are presented. In most cases, the parents have noticed that the child is slow to talk in *any* language, and they seek help for language development. We must rely on them to translate the words and gestures that the child is using and to help us figure out how to build treatment strategies into their everyday life. In these cases we certainly learn as much from them as they do from us since our knowledge about ethnic differences is enhanced.

The cultural differences that have affected our work relate to families whose understanding of "family" is very different from ours. We learned to respect the foster mother who was the center of a large extended family that included brothers, sisters, parents, cousins, nieces and nephews. When she was unable to attend a session because a family member needed her help, we responded with genuine admiration for her ability to juggle her many responsibilities. She was unfailingly creative and helpful whenever she was able to meet with us, and our respect for her led to a strong partnership even though she had been labeled uncooperative and uncaring by other professionals who interacted with her. In another case, the "family" included neighbors and friends who wandered in and out of the apartment during our home visits; some spoke a language unfamiliar to us, but familiar to the child in question. Even with the help of a translator we were unable to figure out if these folks were related to one another but did yearn for a similar support system in our own daily lives! The principles and procedures of Family-Based Treatment are ideally suited to working with families whose ethnicity and culture is different from ours.

Cognitive Differences

Some of our clients show cognitive deficits and, in many cases, one or more family members show similar deficits. Allison was born with hydrocephaly. Her speech and language were slow to develop, and she had facial differences very similar to those of her mother Susan. Her father, step-father James and half-brother Christopher did not show facial differences but both seemed to have difficulty processing information. Susan reported that Allison's father did not complete eighth grade. The clinician slowed her rate of speech, spoke in simple sentences and commented on the caring love that both parents demonstrated to their children.

Susan seemed reluctant to talk and appeared to be very uncomfortable with the one-way mirror that was being used. The clinician, sensitive to this, suggested that she sit in a chair with her back to the mirror. Gradually, as the clinician learned about Susan and James's desires for their daughter, and identified speech-language strategies that they could use, both parents warmed to the process. The clinician wondered if these parents may have been fearful that they wouldn't understand what was being done for their daughter or that they would be criticized for their down-to-earth style. They became helpful partners in treatment and, in fact, reminded us of the power and beauty of simplicity.

Adults who are developmentally disabled can teach the clinician to slow down, identify small steps, and to develop workable solutions that can be used by them and their caregivers. They also teach us to remember to play as did two of our clients. We accompanied them, one diagnosed with Down Syndrome and the other with mental retardation and Tourettes Syndrome to a minor-league baseball game. Parents and residential facility staff appreciated the respite that the outing provided. Our clients showed us how to really enjoy a good ball game by delighting in every aspect of the experience. Communication opportunities were enhanced in the context of an experience that was fun for clinicians and clients alike.

Emotional Differences

Emotional differences may be among the most challenging situations that clinicians encounter. Family members and clients don't always show their emotions in obvious ways, and the clinician may be unclear about what is being expressed. If the clinician is uncomfortable with expressions of feeling, it may be hard to recognize, let alone reflect, the emotions being expressed. Or, if the clinician feels attacked, particularly if family members' statements are negative reactions to the services he is providing, it can be difficult to respond empathically.

Peter's mother, Mary Jo, arrived at our sixth session with her family in tow. She appeared to be unhappy and showed signs of crabbiness and unrest. Our first reaction when she asked, in a disgruntled voice, for more testing to be done was that she must be disappointed with the work that we had been doing and did not favor systemic treatment. We didn't know that Mary Jo was dealing with a developmental transition that had thrust her into the realization that Peter, who had Down Syndrome, would never be "typical." Fortunately, instead of responding defensively to her emotional state, we remembered to ask in a respectful way what had happened when the family tried the assignment that had been suggested two weeks earlier. Mary Jo replied that they didn't have time to do the assignment because she had been busy visiting several kindergarten classrooms in order to make a decision about Peter's placement. We abandoned our efforts to discuss assignments and used neutral questions, clarification and reflection to help us understand her situation. It became clear that Mary Jo was experiencing renewed grieving that had come to the fore as she observed normally developing children in the classroom. We acknowledged her sadness, sat quietly with her as she and her husband reflected on their situation and then told her that we would be happy to do some additional testing. She said that she didn't really need new testing but was terribly worried about how Peter would handle the mainstreamed classroom that he would be entering in three months. We reflected her concern and asked if she would like us to meet with her and the kindergarten teacher, in the placement she selected, to discuss speech-language goals for the school setting. She brightened, showed relief and said, "Yes!"

Our intent in listening to Mary Jo's concerns was *not* to try to stop her from feeling bad. We listened because we knew that she needed a caring ear during a difficult transition. In this case, the listening also led to a way to be helpful, but we would not want the reader to assume that this is always the case. Grieving shows up in many different ways. It's expression cannot be predicted and requires a response that is idiosyncratic to the situation and to the clinician's own comfort with the emotions being expressed. Often, we have been startled by tears, sullenness, unusual quietness and/or anger that appears unexpectedly in our sessions. We, our students, and our colleagues are very relieved to know that respect, caring and reflection make it possible for us to gain at least a small understanding of the emotions that are being expressed. Paradoxically, the situation seems to become less frightening for our clients and for us when this kind of listening is used. If the reader would like to experiment with this technique, try using respect, clarification and reflection with a friend or family member who is experiencing sadness. It is very likely that the friend will become calmer and will gain insight into her situation. The situation will not change, but the presence of an understanding listener will make it easier to bear. Also, it is quite likely that the listener's relationship with the friend will be strengthened.

An emotion that can be particularly difficult to deal with is anger, particularly when it is directed at the clinician or at some aspect of her clinical work. Anger is a secondary emotion that is expressed when a primary emotion is being felt. For example, feelings of failure, hopelessness, abandonment, fear, or sadness may be experienced, but what is shown is anger. Jack's family confronted the clinician with an angry response when they learned that the services they wanted could not be provided. The clinician decided to reflect the feelings that she thought might be part of the angry statements by responding with, "You're very upset with me because the intensive services you want cannot be arranged." To which a parent responded, "Oh, no, we're not upset with you; we're upset with the system that cannot support what we want. Later, the clinician said, "You're worried that your precious Jack's full potential won't be realized without the intense treatment that you want him to have." The reader must remember that listening is not agreeing (Chapter 8), and though family members may show anger and disappointment, reflective responses let them know that the clinician has empathy for their situation. The clinician, in this case, followed up with an I-statement, "I'm really sorry that I can't provide the services you want. May I call you next week to check in and see how things are going? You can always contact me, too, if you decide to continue working with me as a family."

Tears may accompany a variety of clinical situations and signal deep sorrow. Paul, a fifty-seven-year old accountant suffered a stroke that affected his cognition, speech, language and physical abilities. He attended sessions with his wife of thirty-five years. Tears, which were organically as well as emotionally based, were present in many of his early sessions. The clinician listened empathically as Paul found words and gestures to describe his frustration. As he felt heard and as treatment was modified to meet his needs, the tears subsided and were not longer present by the fourth meeting. Reflective listening, which can include silence as well as words, is always appropriate when grief is shown through tears.

Conversational Style Differences

Here we will describe two differences that may call for the use of an I-statement. A situation that we have encountered, though infrequently, is when a parent fills the treatment session with talk, leaving little room for the clinician to offer suggestions for change. As we have stated, we like to listen carefully to our clients and their family members to assure a full understanding of their perspectives about the problem, to identify their resources, and to establish an equal partnership. When the family members' expressions become repetitive, focused almost totally on themselves rather than on opportunities for speech-language change, and we find ourselves becoming frustrated with the situation, we may use an I-statement. The solution-focused principle "if it doesn't work do something different" guides our thinking in these situations (see Chapter 1).

For example, a mother we worked with was dealing with the realization that her son's speech and language difficulties were undoubtedly associated with an autism spectrum disorder. She and her husband were also in the process of divorcing, though both parents regularly attended Family-Based Treatment sessions. Occasionally her former husband was not able to attend scheduled sessions, and at those sessions the mother chatted non-stop about her son and his situation. The clinician guessed that the mother needed to express her feelings in order to release resources to effectively help her son. After three sessions of respectful listening, however, the clinician began to feel uncomfortable because none of the talk focused on the child's communication needs. The clinician decided to try an I-statement and said, "I'm beginning to feel uncomfortable (she began with "I" and then stated her feeling) because we haven't focused on Evan's speech and language for several sessions now (description of the situation). Would it be all right with you if we spent the next thirty minutes discussing his responses to the activities you have been doing with him (request for change)? The mother responded by saying, "Of course, I hadn't realized that we were getting off track." At the end of the session, the clinician and mother decided to spend about fifteen minutes, each session, "catching up" and planned to devote the last thirty-five minutes of each meeting to the child's communication and jointly planned assignments.

Another situation we have occasionally encountered is when a family member appears to be disinterested in the treatment process. One of our very competent graduate students was meeting for the first time with the child of a solo mother who brought a magazine into the treatment room and proceeded to read it, seemingly disinterested in the child's situation. The clinician realized that magazine reading may occur as a part of medical model treatment when the parent is not invited to participate, that the mother may have viewed treatment as a time for a brief respite, or that the mother did not know that her participation was desired. With some trepidation, the clinician decided to use an I-statement and said, "I know from experience that I'll be much more effective as I work with your son if you could help me learn more about him. Would you be willing to answer a few questions so that I can decide how best to assess his situation?" Notice that the clinician used language that was likely to fit the parent's reality (framed in medical model language). She hoped that as she asked open questions and began using solution-focused tracking to understand the mother's concerns that joining would take place. In this case, the mother put her magazine down and participated in the assessment conversation though she never became fully partnered with the clinician. She did, however, attend sessions regularly and usually responded when the clinician requested her input.

Parenting Style Differences

One of the most difficult differences to negotiate is when a family's interactive/ disciplinary style is very different from the clinician's beliefs about what would be best for the client. Angela was a child in such a family, and the clinician needed to muster an extra measure of patience and respect in order to help Angela gain speech-language competence.

Angela's, young mother Jennifer, her grandmother Sue, and her great-grandmother Beatrice all functioned as Angela's parents and had similar disciplinary styles. Their patterns of interaction had likely evolved over several generations and were characterized by rapid-fire questions (which Angela did not answer, responding instead with temper outbursts), critical and demeaning comments about Angela's behavior, obvious discomfort with the clinician's attempts to highlight family resources, and rather constant complaining about the day-care setting that Angela attended. The clinician was certain that if he criticized Angela's parents he would be doing "more of the same" instead of introducing news of difference into their system. He also knew that long-standing family patterns are more likely to change if the clinician models another way of interacting rather than lecturing the family about changes they must make. Therefore, he used clarification, reflection, and solution-focused tracking in order to promote the partnership process; continued to compliment the parents and Angela on small changes that they made; modeled an alternate way of interacting with Angela by following her lead and encouraging her use words and phrases that she could say perfectly; and visited Angela's day-care center to consult with the staff in order to offer suggestions for speech-language interaction with Angela.

Angela's situation was *extremely* challenging as the family's interaction with her changed very little. The clinician found himself hoping that the family might cancel a session from time-to-time, but they faithfully showed up for every scheduled session. Over a six month period Angela's developing speech-language competence, small positive changes in the parents' interaction with Angela, and the support of colleagues gave the clinician the energy he needed to continue his work with the family. At last, the clinician felt that a partnership had developed, even though differences continued to exist. A colleague who had been sharing the clinician's frustration said, "Just *tell* them not to ask so many questions!" and the clinician decided to suggest that the family not ask Angela questions.

The clinician decided to frame the assignment as a challenge: "I have a suggestion, but it's something that's very difficult to do. I'll tell you what it is, and you can decide if you want to try it. The suggestion is to avoid asking any questions and instead make only statements to Angela. What do you think?" This was followed by discussion, demonstration as the clinician played with Angela for a few minutes, and by practice by the parents. Surprisingly, the family made a game of the technique, mockingly cajoling anyone who asked a question as they practiced. The assignment appeared to have been accepted as the family put their own "spin" on it. The next several sessions included joking stories about times that a family member had asked a question! If the clinician had made this suggestion early in treatment it would probably have been rejected but, surprisingly, the family agreed to the suggestion even though the notion of not asking questions still seemed quite strange to them. The clinician's trust in the family and in himself paid off since they were able to follow-through, and a somewhat different style of interacting began to take hold. Angela began using intelligible words in two and three word sentences thus rewarding her parents' efforts. They continued to reject the clinician's compliments, perhaps showing a cultural belief that one should not think too highly of oneself. However, Angela's speech-language improved and tantrums stopped accompanying the family to treatment. This family's love for their child, and their unspoken respect for the clinician, kept them actively engaged in the process even though the clinician had some "strange" ideas.

Family members often show interactive styles different from the clinician's. Though rare, we have worked with husbands who ordered their wives around, and wives who followed those orders (a style that would definitely not work for us!), mothers whose style seems more suitable to the marines than to family life (not particularly useful from our perspective), family members who showed disdain for the treatment process (how can they possibly not enjoy a process that gives *us* so much enjoyment?), and fathers who refused to play with their children (unlike Jim, who plays with such abandon that families may wonder what has happened to his dignity). These families appear to be comfortable with the style that they have adopted even though it is different from ours. We do not try to change their style unless it is interfering with speech-language change as in Angela's case or if abuse and neglect is evident (more about that later in this chapter).

Clinical Procedure Differences

Most of our families are involved in Family-Based Treatment because they have chosen it over the individual model. This fact, as well as our partnership approach, may account for the fact that nearly all of our clients and families fully support the clinical goals and procedures that we jointly develop. We have experienced few, though noteworthy, exceptions to this rule and will now describe our responses to these exceptions.

Some family members do not experience the communicative disorder as a problem and do not understand why they have been referred for services. When this is the case, we ask them to describe the referring person's concerns, and we track family member's responses to those concerns. We also do an assessment with family participation to determine whether we believe that the client could benefit from speech-language services. We describe what we notice during the assessment (see Chapter 3) and, if the client falls within the normal range, we suggest that the family call us if, sometime in the future, they become concerned about the client's communication. We often ask if it would be all right for us to give them a call in a few months to "see how things are going." Family members relax when their perspective is respected and confirmed and leave the session feeling enabled to make decisions. Since change is happening all the time, and we have signaled our ability to work with them as partners, they are more likely to call us in the future if the need arises.

If the assessment indicates to us that treatment would be wise, we ask the family members if they would be willing to work with us to satisfy the referring person or others who are concerned about the child's speech. We do not tell them that *they* should be concerned. Instead, we acknowledged their ability to communicate effectively with the client. In almost every case the family is willing to work with us because we have framed the situation accurately; it is a concern for others but not for them. Grandparents, educators, neighbors, physicians, child protection workers, and early intervention specialists are among those who may have expressed concern about the client's speech-language. If the family members are willing, we invite those persons to one or more sessions to help us better understand their concerns. If this is not possible, the family and client (if over age twelve) usually gives us permission to contact the referring person. The key to the success of this intervention is that we really do not want to try to force the family to deny their communicative competence. In fact, we want them to use that competence to help others who are concerned about the client.

Clinicians who work in other settings have told us that occasionally a family will refuse treatment of any kind. In these cases, we recommend that the clinician remind herself that the family, not she, is ultimately responsible for the child and has the right to accept or refuse services. The clinician should listen carefully and respectfully as the family member describes her reasons for declining treatment, thus creating a safe place for speaking one's mind. The person can then be encouraged to call the clinician again if sometime in the future she would like to discuss possibilities for treatment. When the door is left open for future contact, both the family and the clinician can feel that they are doing the best job possible.

When family members ask the clinician to do something that she cannot do because the request seems unethical to her, she should use a gentle, empathic I-Statement to explain her position. Most families, though disappointed, will accept her explanation. An example of this that speech-language clinicians are unlikely to encounter, is when child protective services must be contacted due to child abuse and neglect. I (Mary) in my family therapy practice almost always let the family know that I must make the call. I express regret that the call may create additional stress for the family but that I am ethically bound to report. The therapeutic partnership is usually not broken, even in very trying circumstances, when direct honesty is used.

INSIDE THE FAMILY CHALLENGES

When family members are conflicted about issues unrelated to speech-language problems, these conflicts can reverberate throughout the treatment system. One cannot ignore the tension associated with couple differences, child behavior problems, or child abuse and neglect. These families unintentionally interject their differences into the treatment process in a powerful way, and we must remember to "do something different" in order to achieve the speech-language change that the family and clinician want.

Couple Conflict

When parents are divorcing, a child benefits from contact with both parents and their agreement about decisions that affect the child. Speech-language pathologists, audiologists, educators and others who work with children are in an excellent position to assure that conflict is minimized by including both parents in decision-making processes. This is not an option, of course, in those rare instances when a parent has been ordered by the court to have no contact with the child.

Justin's mother, Bonnie, was referred to our Clinic following a pre-school screening report of delayed speech and language. During the convening phone call she said that she did not want her estranged husband to attend Family-Based Treatment sessions even though the parents had arranged shared custody. The clinician explained that our sessions include all family members who spend time with the child and who are concerned about the child's speech and language, even if the parents are divorcing. Bonnie agreed to invite her estranged husband, Bob, to the session but said that he would not be much help. The family arrived for the first session, entered the treatment room, and the clinician recognized that anger and resentment, though not invited, had also joined the session. Justin, however, appeared to be delighted to have his parents there and played happily with his father while his mother described the speech-language difficulties that Justin was experiencing. Both parents were excellent sources of information and participated together in the clinical assessment. Bob followed Justin's lead as they played, repeated Justin's phrases to clarify what he was saying and expanded on Justin's one-word utterances. Bonnie asked Justin to say certain words, in order to help the clinician's gain an understanding of the difficulties he was having. The parents did not speak to one another but followed the clinician's lead as they focused on strategies they both could use to help Justin communicate more effectively. The clinician experienced the animosity the parents felt for one another but steadfastly continued to include both parents as treatment partners.

About two months later, the clinician was surprised to see another man in the waiting area whom Bonnie introduced as her boyfriend. Bob had arrived earlier and was also in the waiting room. Since Bonnie invited her friend to join them in the session, the clinician suggested that he observe the session rather than actively participate. The boyfriend appeared to be relieved that he could adopt the role of an observer. Using "use of self" (see Chapter 8), the clinician listened to her personal feelings about the situation and recognized that she would not be able to continue to help Justin since increased animosity had come to treatment with the friend and likely would interfere with the clinician's ability to help Justin. She decided to "do something different" and met with the parents alone to ask if they would like to each attend every-other-week so that they each would have a session alone with their son. Both parents readily agreed, and a new treatment system was formed. Once the new system was formed, the friend discontinued attending, and Bonnie brought Justin's grandmother to her sessions thus expanding the resources that were used to assist Justin.

The reader might ask why the clinician did not meet separately with the parents from the outset. This certainly would have been an option. We have found, however, that if we meet with both parents, for at least a few sessions, we have a better understanding of the child's situation and have established clear access to both parents without becoming triangulated between them. This arrangement can be unsettling at first, but we believe that the best interest of the child is served when the clinician has free access to the people who are most important in his life.

In the unlikely event that adult family members quarrel with one another in the session, the clinician can consider the following responses. First, let the quarrel play itself out and end naturally. The clinician can get back to business when the quarrel has ended. Some families "fight for fun," and they may be showing the clinician one of their interactive differences. If the quarrel doesn't run down on its own, or if it is frequently repeated and treatment is affected, the clinician can use clarification and reflection to listen first to one and then to the other quarreling family member. This is particularly useful when their differences relate to the communication problem of a family member. As the clinician listens, the quarreling members will experience the other family member's views in a more detached and perhaps different way. Simultaneously the clinician will gain a better understanding of their differences which she may want to reframe in a both/and perspective. If neither of these strategies works, the clinician can use an I-statement such as, "I feel uncomfortable as I listen to you argue (the clinician's feeling about the situation) because I'm afraid we won't have enough time, here, to make decisions about how to help Justin. Would it be all right with you if we work together with Justin to help him communicate more effectively ?" (request for change). Family involvement is always focused on enhancing speech language change, and the counseling techniques are integrated, at appropriate times, to assist the clinician and family as they focus on those concerns. There is, however, no set formula that can be used in every case when internal family conflict appears in the session. A caring, respectful clinician who uses counseling techniques will usually be able to figure out what to do. We often remind ourselves that we don't know the solution to every challenge, but we are confident that one will eventually emerge from a partnered relationship.

When family members are conflicted about the care that should be provided to an adult member of their family, and all members are not able to participate in treatment due to travel distances, it is best to try to gather everyone together at least once to develop goals and treatment strategies. The clinician then knows that everyone is "in on" the plans that have been made. When she receives a call from a family member, she can refer back to the family meeting and, if confusion begins to reassert itself, can request another meeting. Most conflict is exacerbated by conversations that do not include all of the concerned family members. Conflict can be resolved, at least in part, when family members discuss directly with one another what they want for their member who is disabled. A respectful, caring clinician can facilitate this process.

Behavior Challenges

Adults, as well as children, can show behavior challenges during speech-language treatment sessions. An adult who has suffered a stroke or a head injury may lash out in ways that are atypical of the person's premorbid personality. I (Mary) worked with an adult client whose speech had been severely affected as a result of a head injury. The client became angry and sometimes verbally abusive with his wife and daughter when they didn't understand his speech. I used solution-focused tracking with the client, his wife, and his adult daughter to identify times that his speech was easiest (not perfect, just easiest!) to understand. They all agreed that when the television and radio were off, when they were looking directly at one another, and when the client was rested, understanding was better. A noticing assignment, designed to gather more information about their most successful interactions, revealed that when the client repeated his statements at least twice and when one-on-one conversations occurred, more understanding ensued. The client and his family members adopted these strategies, and the temper outbursts decreased.

When working with children and their families, we do not want to usurp the parental role, so we provide plenty of opportunities for parents to discipline their children. Interestingly, most difficulties seem to be associated with the way we organize the therapy room. Too many toys, stray cords and plugs, using treatment tools that are not developmentally appropriate, and our huge observation mirror that some children delight in pounding create the greatest challenges. We have the unfortunate/good-fortune (this is an intended both/and phrase) to have a VCR monitor in each of our large therapy rooms. Children gravitate toward the camera like little magnets, and most parents are able to let children know that the camera is off limits. In the rare event that a parent allows the child to "play" with the camera, we ask if would be all right if we remove the child from the tempting situation. By asking the parents if would be all right, we are supporting the hierarchy by letting the parents know that their word is final. We always ask permission before we intervene and have used the phrase "would it be all right" in a variety of situations. Parents always say "yes" as they are as stymied by out-of-bounds behavior as we are and are grateful for our assistance.

We try our behavior management strategy with the child once we have been given permission by the parents to do so. If it is successful, we might say something like, "Whew, that worked this time. Maybe I got lucky. What do you think of that way of responding to him?" This lets the parents know that the child's behavior is challenging, our success was not meant to show them up and again asks them to be the final authorities on the usefulness of the technique. If our attempt is unsuccessful, it provides an excellent opportunity for joining with the parents by saying, "Well, that didn't work. I can sure understand how challenging it is to figure out how to help Johnny learn to control his behavior." Parents feel respected when the clinician acknowledges that their task is a difficult one.

Another technique that we use is to wait for an appropriate interaction to occur and then amplify that behavior. For example, commenting on how cooperative the child is when gently cradled in his mother's lap, noticing that the child calms down when her father speaks in a quiet voice, commenting on how helpful a sibling is when he joins the child in an interesting activity, and commenting on the way a wife's patience and love for her husband creates an environment in which the successful interactions are likely to be repeated.

When the interactions observed in sessions seem to be exacerbating the speech-language problem, we model a different way of interacting with the client. This is done as a natural part of assessment and treatment and is intermingled with conversations about speech-language change. It is never our intent to try to convince family members that they are doing something wrong. Rather, we hope to create a new way of interacting that is effective enough to pique the family members' interest. For example, if a family member talks for an adult client who is capable of speaking for himself, during our next interaction with the client we model slow speech, turn-taking and other behaviors that show respect for and confidence in the client. When we interact differently with children, we never say, "See, that worked a lot better. Why don't you try that at home." Rather, we say, "When I tried following Johnny's lead, he responded a little bit better." Often, parents begin interacting differently with the child after they observe the clinician's model. Their interest is piqued because they experience enhanced client communicative competence resulting from the new interaction.

Family Violence

Speech-language pathologists and audiologists are mandated reporters of child abuse and neglect in most states. When the clinician has first-hand knowledge of abuse or neglect, the child protective services hot-line for the state must be called. The professional who takes the call will be able to determine if the reported situation should be investigated. Cases that are investigated are either "founded" or "unfounded." If founded, the local courts will decide if the child should be removed from the home or if services should be offered to the family while the child remains in the home. The clinician will not be part of the court process though, in some states, she may be asked to file a confidential report and may be interviewed by child protective services as part of the investigation process.

If a client reveals spouse abuse, she should be referred to the nearest shelter program for counseling and advice. The clinician can have phone numbers available for shelter services as well as other area counseling services should such a referral become necessary. We have never had to make a referral like this in our Family-Based Treatment practice but have worked with clients who were receiving services from shelter programs. Adults who are disabled are especially vulnerable to abuse and may need assistance in seeking these services. Elder abuse may also occur, and the area agency on aging can provide information about the client's legal rights and services that are available to assist her.

In almost every case involving family violence, the clinician should continue to work with the client and the family, even when the clinician is the person who reports the abuse. The abusive individual has probably encountered personal abuse at some point in life and will have difficulty changing if the rehabilitative system continues to treat him in a disrespectful, abusive manner. Fortunately, the speech-language pathologist or audiologist will not be assigned the task of helping the individual change his or her abusive behavior; that will be the job of other well-trained professionals. Also, the client's speech-language needs continue, and the family will benefit from the continuing support of a caring professional during what is sure to be a very stressful time.

SUMMARY

Family-Based Treatment naturally involves some challenging family situations though, in the authors' experience, these are rare. When they do arise, however, the clinician has many options. When the clinician is patient, respectful of differences, uses counseling techniques, sets clear boundaries, and has supportive colleagues she is likely to respond well even when the situation is quite stressful. Many challenging situations are associated with differences in perspective between the clinician and the family members. When the clinician shows respect, understanding, non-judgmental listening, and a solution-focus, these differences will be less formidable. When challenges result from factors inside the family, such as divorce conflicts, out-of-bounds behavior, or abuse and neglect, several strategies can be employed to ease the treatment situation. Central to working with all of these challenges is the clinician's trust in herself and her own good judgment, an ability to respect each family member's perception of the situation, and to stay focused on creating speech-language change.

BIBLIOGRAPHY

Anderson S., Russell, C. & Schumm, W. (1983). Perceived marital quality and family life cycle categories: A further analysis. *Journal of Marriage and the Family, 45*, 127-139.

Andrews, J. & Andrews, M. (1986a). A short-term family systems approach to speech-language treatment as a supplement to school-based services. *Seminars in Speech and Language, 7*, 407-414.

Andrews, J. & Andrews, M. (1986b). A family-based systemic model for speech-language services. *Seminars in Speech and Language, 7*, 359-365.

Andrews, M. (1986). Application of family therapy techniques to the treatment of language disorders. *Seminars In Speech and Language, 7*, 347-358.

Andrews, M.A. and Andrews, J.R. (1993). Family-centered techniques: Integrating enablement into the IFSP process. *Journal of Childhood Communication Disorders, 15*, 41-46.

Andrews, J. & Andrews, M. (1995). Solution-focused assumptions that support family-centered intervention. *Infants & Young Children, 8*, 60-67.

Bateson, G. (1979). *Mind and nature*. New York: Dutton.

Benjamin, A. (1981). *The helping interview*. Boston: Houghton Mifflin.

Berg, I.K. (1994). Family based services: *A solution-focused approach*. New York: W.W. Norton.

Bruce, M., DeVenere, N. & Bergeron, C. (1998). Preparing students to understand and honor families as partners, *American Journal of Speech-Language Pathology*, 7, 85-94.

Burr. W. (1972). Role transitions: A reformulation of theory. *Journal of Marriage and the Family, 34*, 407-416.

Butler, W. & Powers, K. (1996).Solution-focused grief therapy. In S.C. Miller, M.A. Hubble & B.L. Duncan (Eds.), *Handbook of solution-focused brief therapy.* (pp. 228-247). San Francisco: Jossey Bass.

Burns, M.S. (1996). Use of the family to facilitate communicative changes in adults with neurological impairments. *Seminars in Speech and Language, 17*, 115-122.

Carter, E.A. & McGoldrick, M. (1980). The family life cycle and family therapy: An overview. In E.A. Carter and M. McGoldrick (Eds.), *The family life cycle: A framework for family therapy* (pp. 3-20). New York: Gardner Press, Inc.

Crais, E.R. (1991). Moving from "parent involvement" to family-centered services. *American Journal of Speech-Language Pathology, 1*, 5-8.

Crais, E.R. and Leonard, C. (1990). P.L. 99-457: Are speech-language pathologists prepared for the challenge? *ASHA, 33*, 57-61.

DeJong, P. & Berg, I.K. (1998). *Interviewing for Solutions.* Pacific Grove, CA: Brooks/Cole Publishing.

Dell, P. F. (1982). Beyond homeostasis: Toward a concept of coherence. *Family Process, 21*, 21-41.

DePompei, R. (1987). A systems approach to understanding CHI family functioning. *Cognitive Rehabilitation, March/April, 1987*, 6-10.

deShazer, S. (1988). *Clues: Investigating solutions in brief therapy.* New York: W.W. Norton.

deShazer, S. (1985). *Keys to solution in brief therapy.* New York: W.W. Norton.

deShazer, S. (1982). Some conceptual distinctions are more useful than others. *Family Process, 21*, 71-84.

Donahue-Kilburg, G. (1992). *Family-centered early intervention for communication disorders.* Gaithersburg, MD: Aspen.

Duncan, B.L., Hubble, M.A. & Miller, S.C. (1997). *Psychotherapy with "impossible" cases.* New York: W.W. Norton.

Dunst, C., Johanson, C., Trivette, C. and Hamby, D. (1991) Family-oriented early intervention policies and practices: Family-centered or not? *Exceptional Children, 58*, 115-126.

Dunst, C., Trivette, C., & Deal, A. (1988). *Enabling and empowering families: Principles and guidelines for practice.* Cambridge, MA: Brookline Books.

Duvall, E. M. (1977). *Family development. (5th Ed.).* Philadelphia: Lippincott.

Dyer, E. (1963). Parenthood as crisis: A restudy. *Marriage and Family Living, 25*, 196-201.

Ellis, L., Schlaudecker, C., & Regimbal, C. (1995) Effectiveness of a collaborative consultation approach to basic concept instruction with kindergarten children. *Language, Speech, and Hearing Services in Schools, 26*, 69-74.

Epstein, N. & Bishop, D. (1981). Problem centered systems therapy of the family. In A. S. Gurman & D. P. Kniskern (Eds.), *Handbook of family therapy* (pp. 444-482). New York: Brunner/Mazel.

Fehsenfeld, D., Andrews, J., Smart, L., Andrews, M. & Wark, L. (1996). Parents reactions to participation in family-centered speech-language services. Poster Session presented at the Annual Meeting of the American Speech-Language-Hearing Association, Seattle, WA.

Fenson, L., Dale, P., Reznick, S., Thal, D., Bates, E., Hartung, J., Pethick, S., & Reilly, J. (1993) *The Macarthur Communicative Development Inventories.* San Diego, CA: Singular Publishing.

Fisch, R., Weakland, J. H. & Segal, L. (1982). *The tactics of change.* San Francisco: Jossey Bass.

Fleuridas, C., Nelson, T. and Rosenthal, D. (1986). The evolution of circular questions: Training family therapists. *Journal of Marital and Family Therapy, 12*, 113-127.

Fortier, L. & Wanlass, R. L. (1984). Family crisis following the diagnosis of a handicapped child. *Family Relations, 33*, 3-24.

Frassinelli, L., Superior, K. & Meyers, J. (1983). A consultation model for speech and language services. *ASHA, 25*, 25-30.

Garbee, F. (1982). The speech-language pathologist as a member of the educational team. In R.J. Van Hattum (Ed.), *Speech-Language Programming in the Schools* (pp.72-115). Springfield, IL: Charles C. Thomas Publisher.

Gehart-Brooks, D.R. & Lyle, R.R. (1999, January). What works in therapy: Client's perspectives. *Family Therapy News, 29*, p. 25.

Glenn, N. (1975). Psychological well-being in the post-parental stage: Some evidence from national surveys. *Journal of Marriage and the Family, 37*, 105-110.

Goetz, N. (1982). Parental perspectives and concerns. *Seminars in Speech, Language and Hearing, 3*, 274-279.

Hahn, E. (1979). Directed home training program for infants with cleft lip and palate. In K.R. Bzoch (Ed.), *Communicative disorders related to cleft lip and palate* (pp. 311-317). Boston: Little, Brown and Company.

Haley, J. (1987). *Problem solving therapy*. San Francisco: Jossey-Bass.

Haley, J. (1973). *Uncommon therapy*: The psychiatric techniques of Milton H. Erickson, M.D. New York: Norton.

Hofstadter, D. (1979). *Godel, Escher, Bach: An eternal golden braid*. New York: Basic Books.

Johnson, B., McGonigel, M. & Kaufmann, R. (Eds.). (1989). *Guidelines and recommended practices for the individualized family service plan*. Chapel Hill, N.C.: NEC*TAS.

Kresheck. J. & Werner, E. (1989). *Structured Photographic Articulation Test featuring Dudsberry*. DeKalb, IL: Janelle Publications, Inc.

LeMasters, E. (1957). Parenthood as crisis. *Marriage and Family Living,19*, 352-355.

Lewis. M. & Butler, R. (1974). Life review therapy. *Geriatrics, 29*, 165-173.

Long, G. (1990). Introduction. In Long, G. & Harvey, M. (Eds.), *Facilitating the transition of deaf adolescents: Focus on families.* (pp. 1-9). Little Rock, AR: Research and Training Center on Deafness and Hearing Impairment.

Luterman, D. (1996). *Counseling persons with communicative disorders and their families.* Austin, TX: Pro-Ed.

Manolson, A., (1985). *It takes two to talk: A Hanen early language parent guide book.* Toronto: Hanen Early Language Resource Centre.

Madanes, C. (1981). *Strategic family therapy.* San Francisco: Jossey Bass.

McCubbin, H. & Dahl. B. (1985). *Family and marriage: Individuals and life cycles.* New York: John Wiley & Sons.

McGonigel, M.J, Kaufmann, R.K., & Johnson, B.H. (Eds.). (1991). *Guidelines and Recommended Practices for the Individualized Family Service Plan (second edition).* Bethesda, MD: Association for the Care of Children's Health.

Minuchin, S. (1974). *Families and family therapy.* Cambridge: Harvard University Press.

Moses, K. (1985). Dynamic intervention with families. In: *Hearing-impaired children and youth with developmental disabilities: An interdisciplinary foundation for service.* (pp. 82-98) Washington, DC: Gallaudet College Press.

Neidecker, E. (1987). *School programs in speech-language: Organization and management.* Englewood Cliffs: Prentice Hall.

O'Hanlon, W. H. & Weiner-Davis, M. (1989). *In search of solutions.* New York: W. W. Norton, & Co.

Prizant, B. and Meyer, E. (1993). Socioemotional Aspects of Language and Social Communication Disorders in Young Children and Their Families. *American Journal of Speech-Language Pathology, 2*, 56-71.

Rogers, C. (1965). *Client centered therapy*. Boston: Houghton Mifflin.

Rollin, W. J. (1987).*The psychology of communication disorders in individuals and their families*. Englewood Cliffs, New Jersey: Prentice-Hall, Inc.

Rollins, B. & Feldman, H. (1970). Marital satisfaction over the family life cycle. *Journal of Marriage and the Family, 32*, 20-28.

Rossetti, L. (1990). *The Rossetti Infant-Toddler Language Scale*. East Moline, IL: LinguiSystems.

Schwartz, L. (1982). Social services for the family with a cleft palate child. *Seminars in Speech, Language and Hearing, 3*, 268-273.

Scott, S. (1984). Mobilization: A natural resource of the family. In J. C. Hansen & E. I. Coppersmith (Eds.), *Families with handicapped members* (pp. 98-110). Rockville, MD: Aspen Systems Corporation.

Seibel, N. (1987a). A parent's perspective. *The ACPA/CPF Newsletter* (pp. 1-2). American Cleft Palate Association: Pittsburgh, PA.

Seibel, N. (1987b). Untitled. Unpublished manuscript.

Selekman, M. D. (1993). *Pathways to change*: Brief therapy solutions with difficult adolescents. New York: Guilford.

Simon, F., Stierlin, H. & Wynne, L. (1985). *The language of family therapy: systemic vocabulary and sourcebook*. New York: Family Process Press.

Solomon, M. A. (1973). A developmental conceptual premise for family therapy. *Family Process, 12*, 179-188.

Spanbock, P. (1987). Understanding head injury from the families' perspective. *Cognitive Rehabilitation*, March/April, 12-14.

Suelzle, M., & Keenan, V. (1981). Changes in family support networks over the life cycle of mentally retarded persons. *American Journal of Mental Deficiency, 86*, 267-274.

Superior, K. & Lelchook, A. (1986). Family participation in school-based programs. *Seminars in Speech and Language, 7*, 395-404.

Tomm, K. (1984). One perspective on the Milan systemic approach: Part I. Overview of development, theory and practice. *Journal of Marital and Family Therapy,10*, 113-125.

Tomm, K. (1988). Interventive interviewing: Part III. Intending to ask circular, strategic, or reflexive questions. *Family Process, 27*, 1-15.

Vander Zanden, J. W. (1989). *Human development*. New York: Alfred A. Knopf.

Van Riper, C. (1954). *Speech correction: Principles and methods*. Englewood Cliffs, NJ: Prentice-Hall.

Walter, J. & Peller, J. (1992). *Becoming solution-focused in brief therapy*. New York: Brunner/Mazel.

Wilcox, M. J. (1989). Delivering communication-based services to infants,toddlers, and their families: Approaches and models. *Topics in Language Disorders, 10*, 68-79.

Wikler, L., Wasow, M., & Hatfield, E. (1983). Looking for strengths in families of developmentally disabled children. *Social Work, July/August*, 313-315.

Williams, S. C. (1986). Family-focused treatment: A speech-language pathologists role in a home-based parent training program. *Seminars in Speech and Language 7*, 383-393.

Appendix A

FAMILY-BASED TREATMENT
INTAKE FORM

CLIENT'S NAME: _____

Date of Birth: _____ Caller: _____

Mother: _____ Father: _____

Address:_____

_____

Phone: _____

Family Members:_____

_____

_____

Information: _____

_____

_____

_____

Referral Source: _____

_____

First Session: Date _____   Time _____

Appendix B

FAMILY-BASED TREATMENT
CHILD PRE-ASSESSMENT FORM

SPEECH & HEARING CLINIC
NORTHERN ILLINOIS UNIVERSITY
DEKALB, ILLINOIS

Your child has been scheduled for an assessment of his/her speech and language. To help us prepare for your appointment, please complete this form and return it prior to your appointment.

Child's Name: _____ Birthdate: _____

Address: _____ City & State: _____

Parents' Names: _____ Telephone: _____

Other Caregivers (e.g., sitter, grandparents, etc.): _____

Please list the adults who live at home with your child:

_____   _____

_____   _____

Please list the names and ages of other children who live at home with your child:

_____   _____

_____   _____

_____   _____

Please describe your child's speech & language:

_____

_____

_____

_____

Who is concerned about your child's speech & language? _____

_____

_____

What is of most concern? This may differ for different family members so please record all concerns:

_____

_____

_____

Please describe when your child's speech & language is at its best:

_____

_____

_____

What do you and your family members already do to help your child?

_____

_____

_____

What would you like to know about your child's speech & language?

_____

_____

_____

_____

What would you like from this appointment? ————————

_____

_____

<u>On the back of this page</u>, please describe any differences or concerns you have about your child's birth history; medical history/conditions; milestones of physical development like sitting, crawling, standing, walking, etc.; social behavior; academic progress; and/or hearing. What factors do you think are important and may relate to your child's speech and language?

Please return to: Department of Communicative Disorders, Speech & Hearing Clinic, Northern Illinois University, DeKalb, IL 60115.

FAMILY-BASED TREATMENT
ADULT PRE-ASSESSMENT FORM

SPEECH & HEARING CLINIC
NORTHERN ILLINOIS UNIVERSITY
DEKALB, ILLINOIS

You have been scheduled for a speech-language assessment. To help us prepare for your appointment, please complete this form and return it prior to your appointment.

Client's Name: ————————————— Birthdate: ———————————

Address: ————————————— City & State: ——————————

Telephone: ————————————— Physician: ———————————

Please list the adults who live at home with you: _____

_____   _____

_____   _____

Please list the names and ages of any children who live at home with you:

_____   _____

_____   _____

Please describe your speech & language: _____

_____

_____

_____

_____

Who is concerned about your speech & language? _____

_____

_____

_____

_____

What is of most concern? _____

_____

_____

_____

Please describe when your speech & language is at its best:

_____

_____

_____

What do you and/or other family members already do to help you communicate?

_____

_____

_____

What would you like to know about your speech & language?

_____

_____

_____

What would you like from this appointment? _____

_____

_____

_____

If someone referred you for this appointment, please list that person's name:

_____

On the back of this page, please describe any differences or concerns you have about your medical history/conditions, social interactions, hearing, or other factors that relate to your ability to communicate.

Please return to: Department of Communicative Disorders, Speech & Hearing Clinic, Northern Illinois University, DeKalb, IL 60115.

Appendix C

FAMILY-BASED TREATMENT
SESSION NOTES

Client: ————————————————— Date: ——————————————

Participants: (We include names of family members and clinicians)

————————————————————————————————

————————————————————————————————

Comments: ———————————————————————————

————————————————————————————————

(We list compliments that are directly related to speech-language events that occurred during the session, positive speech-language events that were reported in the session by family members, and/or other positive clinician observations. These must be honest comments about actual events that are likely to enable family members to become more actively involved with the client's speech-language change.)

Suggestions: ——————————————————————————

————————————————————————————————

(We list isomorphic assignments that have been created collaboratively during the session)

Next Session: Date ————————————————— Time ——————————

Clinician's Phone number: ————————————————————

INDEX